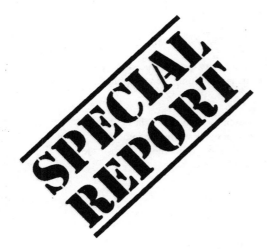

OSTEOPOROSIS:
HOW TO STOP IT
HOW TO PREVENT IT
HOW TO REVERSE IT

ELIZABETH VIERCK

FOR THE 25 MILLION AMERICANS SUFFERING FROM OSTEOPOROSIS, HERE'S A PROVEN PROGRAM TO ALLEVIATE AND REVERSE ITS POTENTIALLY CRIPPLING SYMPTOMS. FOR THE COUNTLESS MILLIONS OF INDIVIDUALS AT RISK, THIS PROGRAM SHOWS HOW TO BUILD STRONGER BONES NOW TO PREVENT OSTEOPOROSIS LATER.

PARKER PUBLISHING COMPANY
West Nyack, New York 10995

This book is a reference work based on research by the author. The opinions
expressed herein are not necessarily those of or endorsed by the publisher.
The directions stated in this book are in no way to be considered as a substitute
for consultation with a duly licensed doctor.

10   9   8   7   6   5   4   3   2   1

Library of Congress Cataloging-in-Publication Data

Vierck, Elizabeth
    Special report : osteoporosis : how to stop it, how to prevent it, how to
reverse it / by Elizabeth Vierck.
       p. cm.
    ISBN 0-13-559782-X
    1. Osteoporosis—Treatment.   2. Osteoporosis—Prevention.   I. Title.
II. Title: Osteoporosis.
    RC931.073V54 1993   93-5849
    616.7'16—dc20   CIP

ISBN 0-13-559782-X

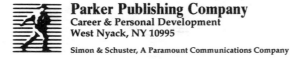

Parker Publishing Company
Career & Personal Development
West Nyack, NY 10995
Simon & Schuster, A Paramount Communications Company

Printed in the United States of America

CONTENTS

<u>INTRODUCTION</u>

<u>WHAT THIS REPORT CAN DO FOR YOU</u>

Why should you read this report? Because you have a one in two chance that by the time you reach age 65 you will have osteoporosis, the "bone thief," which progresses without symptoms and results in broken bones. In addition, if you are young or in your middle years, you have an increasing chance of developing the disease now. You are particularly susceptible if you are an avid athlete, diet frequently, have a medical condition such as small-bowel disease, or take medications such as steroids that block calcium absorption.

Osteoporosis is a common and painful condition that disfigures and disables its victims. It is a disease in which bones become weak and break spontaneously. Its signature is fractures, primarily of the spine, hips, and wrists. Many physical characteristics that we associate with aging, such as a stooped posture, shrinking height, and thick waist are really caused by osteoporosis.

<u>However, the good news is that osteoporosis is preventable if you take the steps spelled out in this</u>

report and continue them throughout your life. And by following the guidelines in this report, you will have increased health and strength. Your heart, bones, and muscles will be strong. You'll have increased energy and endurance. You will look and feel younger.

Many people think of osteoporosis as a condition of older age. Actually, the disease begins in the early adult years, and steps to thwart it should be started then. You can, however, greatly improve your chances against osteoporosis at any age by following the advice in this book. In fact, recent medical studies have shown that, even at age 75, bone mass can be increased significantly through following the steps presented here. The recommendations have been developed and sanctioned by the important medical and research centers that are doing work with victims of the disease, including the National Osteoporosis Foundation and the National Institutes of Health.

Not only does this report explain the major principles and steps for preventing or alleviating osteoporosis, but it also provides tips on what you can do if the steps cannot be followed. For example, the reduction in estrogen that occurs after menopause is strongly linked to the development of osteoporosis in women. However, you may not be able to take estrogen supplements for a medical reason such as a family history of breast cancer. Chapter Six of this report describes alternative treatments that have been found effective in cutting down on bone loss after menopause.

WHO DEVELOPS OSTEOPOROSIS
AND WHAT ARE THE SYMPTOMS?

If you are a woman and are thin, small boned, white, and postmenopausal, you are at extremely high risk for developing osteoporosis. But if you do not fall into this category, you are not risk free. More men, for example, are developing the condition. No matter what your age or sex, if one or more of the following describes you, you are at high risk for developing osteoporosis:

- Poor eating habits and/or an eating disorder

- Do not eat dairy products

- Strenuous dieter and/or faster

- Physically inactive

- Partially or totally immobilized

- Endurance athlete, including running and dancing

- Female and past menopause

- Heavy cigarette smoker

- Heavy drinker of alcohol

- Senior citizen

- Have a medical condition such as small bowel disease or take a medication such as steroids that block calcium absorption.

- A family history of osteoporosis

Unfortunately, osteoporosis usually does not become apparent until significant damage has occurred. It may go undetected until one day you realize that your waist is thicker and you can't diet the excess off and you have lost an inch or two in height. These are permanent changes caused by collapsed vertebrae in the spine.

For victims of osteoporosis, their body weight on their bones causes their spines to compress. Their posture becomes stooped, and they can lose up to eight inches of height. Collapsed vertebrae are also sometimes felt as severe back pain or result in a curvature of the back, called "dowager's hump." On the other hand, sometimes osteoporosis wears away an individual's bones without these characteristics becoming noticeable, until the victim falls and breaks a wrist or hip.

Here are the five most common problems caused by osteoporosis:

1. Loss of height caused by spinal fractures and resulting in a characteristic "aged" appearance with shortened trunk, thick waist, and arms that reach to the knees

2. A humpbacked, round-shouldered posture

3. Hip fractures, often resulting in death

4. Broken wrists

5. Disability

OSTEOPOROSIS—WHAT YOU CAN DO

How can you prevent or alleviate osteoporosis? First, it is important to understand that there is no single special elixir or capsule that you can take that will ward off bone loss. The prevention program that works includes getting the right kind of nutrition and exercise and compensating for health problems that lead to osteoporosis such as low estrogen levels or stomach disorders that block calcium absorption. Briefly, the program involves two major principles:

1. Building up a bone surplus during childhood and the early adult years

2. Maintaining a strong bone structure during older age, when accumulated risk factors can result in osteoporosis.

Both principles involve following four basic steps. Details of these steps follow in Chapters Two through Five. Briefly, the steps are the following:

1. Learn about the risk factors for osteoporosis. The risk factors for osteoporosis have been identified by the important research centers that are doing work on the disease, including the National Osteoporosis Foundation and National Institutes of Health. Learning about these risk factors to take the right steps toward prevention can mean the difference between mobility and disability.

2. Develop a well-rounded, high-calcium nutritional program. When your mother insisted that you drink milk every day to build strong bones, she was

right. Every day, your body naturally loses some calcium, and if it is not replaced, it steals it from your bones. In addition, lack of some foods and vitamins and too much of others interfere with calcium absorption or cause calcium to be lost through the kidneys. Careful attention should be paid to these factors in building a well-rounded nutritional program.

3. Get plenty of weight-bearing exercise. Not getting enough of the right kind of exercise results in bone loss. To slow osteoporosis, the National Institutes on Health recommend at least three to four hours of weight-bearing exercise a week. Brisk walking, running, tennis, and aerobic dance are all weight-bearing activities.

4. Take the appropriate drug therapy as prescribed by a physician. The risk of developing osteoporosis because of a health condition such as menopause can be alleviated by taking the appropriate medication prescribed by your physician. Such medications include hormones, bone builders such as calcitonin, and drugs to treat diseases that cause osteoporosis.

While any of the steps alone will improve your odds against osteoporosis, following all of them maximizes your chances. For example, a study undertaken recently in Australia found that, for women, taking two steps—increasing weight-bearing exercise and calcium intake—cuts down on bone loss. But taking three steps—increasing weight-bearing exercise, maximizing calcium intake, and taking estrogen—enlarges bone density.[1]

There are many benefits that you will achieve from adopting the principles and steps described in this book:

1. You will have strong bones. Your bones will have enough mass and strength to withstand falls or other kinds of accidents.

2. You will avoid disability and pain. Every year 1.3 million people suffer spontaneous fractures because of osteoporosis. In one in five cases of hip fractures the individual dies within three months. You can avoid such fractures and the pain that goes with them.

---

[1] "Bone Savers: Rating Lifestyle and Drugs," Science News, October 21, 1991, p. 262.

3. <u>You will have increased mobility.</u> Because your bones will be strong, you will be able to carry out the physical activities you enjoy despite your age, including snow skiing, tennis, and an active sex life.

4. <u>You will have increased health and strength.</u> The principles and steps in this book will not only give you strong bones, but they will also keep you healthy and give you muscle strength. You'll have more energy and endurance. You will also reduce your risk for heart disease and related problems.

5. <u>You will look and feel younger.</u> You will not have the stooped posture and other characteristics of an aged appearance.

6. <u>If you already have osteoporosis, you can slow its progression.</u> By learning about the risk factors for osteoporosis and taking preventive measures, you will be able to cut down on further bone loss.

7. <u>Because your overall health and appearance will be youthful, you will avoid the depression and isolation that often accompany osteoporosis.</u> Because you will be taking such good care of yourself you will feel better. Exercise, for example, is not only

an important step to osteoporosis prevention, it is also a proven mood elevator. It also cuts down on insomnia and overweight, and reduces pain and stiffness.

By now it should be clear that this special report is important to you if you have any of the risk factors for osteoporosis or if you know someone who does. It is also important to understand that, despite your age, now is the time to make sure you have enough bone in the bank to protect against future losses. The following pages will show how to achieve this and how to avoid the pain and disability that accompany osteoporosis.

CHAPTER ONE

THE BONE THIEF—OSTEOPOROSIS

This special report will show you how to prevent and treat the bone-breaking disease osteoporosis. The statistics speak for themselves: osteoporosis is frighteningly common. One out of two men and women over age 65 is a victim of the disease. The pain and disability of osteoporosis are not confined to senior citizens. Almost a third of the women past age 50 and one-fifth of the men this age are shrinking in height because their spinal columns are crumbling from the disease. Osteoporosis also has the dubious distinction of being the most common health hazard for women past menopause, beating out even arthritis and heart disease.[1] Unhappily, many young people are also developing the condition.

While writing this report I interviewed and read the accounts of men and women of all ages who have been inflicted with osteoporosis. They include the following:

---

[1] Jane Brody, Jane Brody's Nutrition Book, (New York: W. W. Norton, 1981), p. 411.

- A 34-year-old athlete who lost a significant amount of weight at age 31 while she was training for a marathon. Over the next three years she lost an inch of height due to small breaks in her vertebrae. Now she is popping pain killers every four hours for lower-back pain.

- A similar account, reported in the New England Journal of Medicine, of a 22-year-old male marathon runner with poor nutrition, which led to osteoporosis and fractures of the pelvis and the vertebrae.[2]

- A 27-year-old woman who was climbing the stairs one day and heard a loud crack as a sharp pain shot through her lower back. Soon after, her doctor told her that her bones were "like whipped potatoes," the result of years of taking steroids to control a disease called lupus. She now has to wear a brace to support her back.

---

[2] Nancy Rigotti et al., "Osteopenia and Bone Fractures in a Man with Anorexia Nervosa and Hypogonadism," Journal of the American Medical Association, July 18, 1986, pp. 385-388.

- A 45-year-old writer, known as a fun-loving, heavy drinker, whose average alcohol consumption ranged from six to eight drinks a day. He also hated exercise and smoked over a pack of cigarettes a day. The result: severe osteoporosis. Last year, at age 44, he fell and broke his hip while walking his Golden Retriever.

- A grandmother in her eighties who is bedridden. Her bones are so brittle that if she gets up and walks around, she invariably snaps a vertebra.

To learn how to prevent the pain and disability that these people are experiencing, it is helpful to understand what osteoporosis is and how it develops. This information is not necessary to prevent or treat osteoporosis, but it sheds light on how the steps described in this report work and why it is important to follow them.

WHAT IS OSTEOPOROSIS?

The word <u>osteoporosis</u> is derived from the Greek <u>osteon</u> for "bone" and <u>porus</u> for "pore" or "passage." The term was first coined by Fuller Albright in 1940 in a groundbreaking article in the <u>Journal of the American Medical Association</u>, which described much of what we now know to be true about the condition. In short, osteoporosis is a disease in which, over time, bones lose calcium, making them so fragile they break easily, sometimes spontaneously. Left unchecked, the disease results in severe pain, disability, and disfigurement.

The weak bones of osteoporosis are the result of a natural physical process called bone remodeling. Remodeling is your skeleton's way of maintaining strength. Unfortunately, when it goes awry due to poor nutrition, lack of the right kind of exercise, or exposure to other risk factors, the result is weak bones. The following explains bone remodeling and its relationship to the two major principles of osteoporosis prevention.

BONE REMODELING

Bone, like many other body tissues, changes constantly. In fact, it is remarkably active. During remodeling, old bone is torn down, "resorbed," and replaced with new bone in much the same way you would remodel your kitchen by tearing down and replacing walls, cabinets, and floors. Through the remodeling process, bone tissue completely replaces itself every seven years.[3]

───────────────────

[3] David F. Fardon, Osteoporosis, (New York: Macmillan, 1985) p. 47.

Remodeling is always taking place throughout your bone structure. It involves three types of bone cells. <u>Osteoclasts</u> act as demolition crews and remove old bone, <u>osteoblasts</u> act as construction crews and create new bone, and <u>osteocytes</u> maintain the bone structure after it has been remodeled. The entire process is regulated by hormones and takes about four months at each remodeling site.

Osteoporosis occurs when new bone formation and bone loss do not keep up with each other. In other words, developing osteoporosis is like tearing the plaster out of the walls of your kitchen and replacing the material here and there with cardboard, while leaving large holes that are not filled in.

<u>Principle One:</u>
<u>Building a Bone Surplus During Childhood</u>

Osteoporosis is often referred to as a children's issue. Children are bone builders. During childhood, adolescence, and early adulthood, calcium is deposited in bones faster than it is taken out. Bones are gaining strength and density during these years. At about age 35, they reach a point called "peak bone mass." This means that they are as big and sturdy as they will ever be. To put it bluntly, it is a downhill slide from there. They will never be that strong again.

The stage of growth up to your midthirties is very important. Many experts believe that the condition of your bones during this time determines whether you develop weak bones later. This is why the first principle of osteoporosis prevention is to build up a bone surplus during childhood and the early adult years. For example, interfering with the normal production of the female hormone estrogen during this time, through overexercising or strenuous diet, interrupts bone building and results in osteoporosis later.[4]

Principle Two:
Maintain a Strong Bone Structure During Older Age

For unknown reasons, aging depletes bone mass. That is why the second principle of osteoporosis prevention is to maintain a strong bone structure during older age, when accumulated risk factors can result in osteoporosis. Once an individual reaches his or her late thirties, calcium is lost from bones faster than it is replaced.

---

[4] Iris F. Litt, "Adolescent Medicine," Journal of the American Medical Association, June 19, 1991, p. 3101.

Then beginning at age 45 for women and age 60 for men, our bodies also absorb less calcium from food.

These two natural changes result in a net loss of calcium from bones after about age 40. In addition, if any of the risk factors described in the next chapter are present, they further endanger bones. In brief, just a few of these risk factors are decreased estrogen, poor nutrition, lack of weight-bearing exercise, and taking certain medications such as steroids.

BONE STRUCTURE AND OSTEOPOROSIS

Bones are architectural wonders of nature. Their size and shape are determined by genetics, exercise, and gravity. Bones are made up of layers of coiled fibers of protein that make them strong and flexible. Sitting in the crevices of these fibers is calcium salt, which makes them hard. When all is going well, bones are efficient structures, supporting the body.

There are two types of bone. Both change significantly when osteoporosis strikes. Compact or cortical bone is hard and dense. It covers the outside of most bones. Spongy or trabecular bone lies beneath compact bone, consisting of a mesh of open space, bony bars, and bone marrow. Spongy bone is concentrated in the spinal column and at the end of long bones such as the thigh bone. <u>These are the areas of bone that fracture most frequently with osteoporosis.</u>

Beginning in about the midthirties, both men and women lose both types of bone. Cortical bone gets thinner and trabecular bone develops larger spaces. Osteoporosis exaggerates these changes (see Figure 1-1.)

Figure 1-1

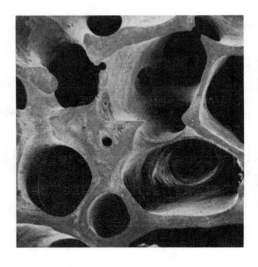 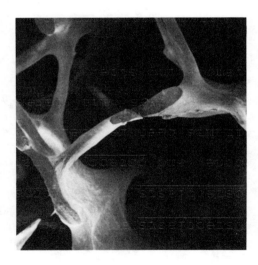

(A) Normal bone   **(B) Osteoporotic bone**

With permission from Dempster et al.,
J. Bone Min Res <u>1</u>, 15-21, 1986.

Each individual's bone structure is unique. Your skeleton's outer shell of cortical bone may be thin and weak, for example, while your sister's is thick and hard. On average, however, over their lifetimes, women lose a third of their cortical bone and men lose one-half.[5] By advanced old age, women lose half their spongy bone and men lose about one-third.[6] A typical 80-year-old woman has lost almost half her spongy bone.[7] When this much trabecular bone is lost bones can break spontaneously.

SIGNS TO WATCH OUT FOR

How can you tell if you have osteoporosis? Unfortunately, it is difficult to detect the disease in the early stages, and your bones may begin crumbling decades before you realize it. The early stages of osteoporosis do not even show up on X rays. Usually, by the time the

---

[5] B. Lawrence Riggs and L. Joseph Melton III, "The Prevention and Treatment of Osteoporosis," New England Journal of Medicine, August 27, 1992, p. 620.

[6] Ibid.

[7] Morris Notelovitz and Marsh Ware, Stand Tall: The Informed Woman's Guide to Preventing Osteoporosis, (Gainesville, FL: Triad, 1982).

disease is detected by medical tests, significant bone is lost. In fact, because spinal fractures can be pain free, it is common to break many vertebrae in the spine long before noticing a problem.

Often the first detectable sign of osteoporosis is loss of height. It is a good idea to measure your height once a year. If you are shrinking, you should see your doctor for an evaluation for osteoporosis. Other signs of osteoporosis are fractures; periodontal disease including changes in the shape of the jaw, receding gums, and loose or shifting teeth; and low-back pain. If you have any of these symptoms, you should see your doctor for an evaluation for osteoporosis.

Fractures:
The Most Damaging Symptom of Osteoporosis

The first sign of osteoporosis is often a broken bone (fracture). Fractures occur in two different ways. Short, fat bones crush; long, cylindrical bones split into pieces and may or may not separate.

Spinal and hip fractures occur most frequently, but breaks may also occur in the ribs, wrist, shoulder, pelvis, or knee joints. (Happily, many other bones, such as the short bones of the hands and feet, the skull, and shoulder blades, are not affected by osteoporosis and are not susceptible to fracture.)

As mentioned earlier, a fractured spine is the signature of osteoporosis, causing the characteristic shrinking and forward thrusting backbone (see Figure 1-2). The spine or backbone includes 33 bones called vertebrae, which are composed primarily of spongy, soft (trabecular) bone. When vertebrae fracture, they collapse in a wedge shape, resulting in a shortened, crippled spine. Fractures occur most often in two points of the spine—where it curves forward and where the ribs end.

Figure 1-2

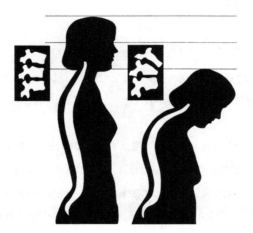

(A) Normal spine   **(B) Fractured spine.**

Source: <u>Stand Up to Osteoporosis</u>, (Washington, D.C.: National Osteoporosis Foundation, Public Information Services) p. 7.

If you fracture a vertebra in your spine, you may feel a sharp pain at the time of the break or no pain at all. Usually, a sharp pain turns into a dull ache that lasts up to a month. Fractures eventually heal, although the bone is permanently disfigured.

Another common problem resulting from osteoporosis is fracturing a hip. If you are a woman, your risk of developing a hip fracture is equal to your <u>combined</u> risk of developing breast, uterine, and ovarian cancer.[8] The lifetime risk of dying from a hip fracture for a 50-year-old woman is equal to the lifetime risk of death due to breast cancer.[9]

---

[8] National Osteoporosis Foundation, "Stand Up to Osteoporosis" (Washington, D.C.: NOF, 1992), p. 10.

[9] S. R. Cummings, et al., "Lifetime Risks of Hip, Colles' or Vertebral Fracture and Coronary Heart Disease Among White Menopausal Women," <u>Archives of Internal Medicine</u>, Vol. 149, 1989, pp. 2445-2448.

Some 300,000 Americans fracture a hip every year, most often because of osteoporosis.[10] A common saying among orthopedic physicians is: "If you break a hip because of osteoporosis, you don't necessarily break it from falling." In other words, first, your bones reach the "fracture threshold," the point where they are so weak they break spontaneously. Then, your hip snaps and you fall down.

Hips usually break in the thinnest part of the thigh bone (the femur). According to the National Osteoporosis Foundation, more than 50 percent of those who fracture a hip lose their ability to walk independently and 30 percent become totally dependent. Fifteen to 20 percent need care in a nursing home, and 12 to 20 percent die within a year.

Fractures of the wrist are also common. Breaks in the lower part of a bone called the radius occur most frequently. Such fractures are called Colles' fractures

---

[10] Steven Cummings et al., "Appendicular Bone Density and Age Predict Hip Fracture in Women," Journal of the American Medical Association, February 2, 1990, p. 665.

and usually happen due to landing on the wrist when trying to break a fall.

TYPES OF OSTEOPOROSIS

There are two major types of osteoporosis. Type I osteoporosis is also called postmenopausal osteoporosis or high-turnover osteoporosis. It is caused by excessive bone demolition and occurs primarily in women between the ages of 51 and 75.[11] Type I osteoporosis can be prevented through hormone therapy. It affects primarily the soft, spongy bone of the spine and forearm.[12]

Type II osteoporosis hits people over age 70. Twice as many women as men develop it. The condition is also called low-turnover osteoporosis, referring to the fact that bone construction is inadequate. Type II osteoporosis affects both the hard outer and soft inner bone of the spine and hips. Fracture sites include the vertebrae, hip, pelvis, and long bones.

---

[11] Barbara Liscum, "Osteoporosis: The Silent Disease," Orthopaedic Nursing, July-August 1992, p. 21.

[12] Angelo A. Licata, "Therapies for Symptomatic Primary Osteoporosis," Geriatrics, November 1991, p. 62.

Osteoporosis resulting from health problems such as gastrointestinal disease or extensive use of medications such as steroids is often referred to by physicians as secondary osteoporosis. It can occur in men or women.

WOMEN AND OSTEOPOROSIS

While men can and do develop osteoporosis, eight times as many women have the disease. There are many reasons for the disparity. Men naturally have larger, denser bones than women and so can afford to lose more bone mass before fractures occur. In addition, women have double jeopardy where osteoporosis is concerned. The natural decrease in estrogen that occurs when fertility stops is a direct cause of Type I osteoporosis (postmenopausal osteoporosis). In addition, both women and men are susceptible to developing Type II osteoporosis, which occurs naturally after age 70, <u>but many more women than men live to this age</u>.

The good news is, for women who can take estrogen, a powerful deterrent to osteoporosis is as far away as the closest prescription counter. Taking estrogen can buy decades of strong and sturdy bones. The bad news, however, is not all women can or should be taking hormones. For detailed information on estrogen and what to do if you cannot take it, see Chapters Five and Six.

ADVANCED OSTEOPOROSIS

Because osteoporosis is a sneaky disease that usually progresses without giving its victim any warning signs, many people do not know they have the condition until it is well advanced. When left unchecked, osteoporosis progresses to a point where appearance and self-esteem are affected. Here is a description of what the bodies of victims of advanced osteoporosis look like:

- The upper body is out of proportion to the arms and legs.

- The victim is usually hunched over and shuffles when he or she walks.

- Often the stomach protrudes. Usually the victim feels awkward and clothes don't fit.

- As the vertebrae collapse, the rib cage tilts downward toward the hips and the upper spine curves outward (called kyphosis).

16

- Because of the changing spine, organs are forced to move to new positions and are often packaged too tightly together. Breathing problems can result and constipation often occurs. Often the rib cage touches the pelvis.

WHAT YOU CAN DO

Osteoporosis is better prevented than treated. To keep careful watch on your bones, it is important to get a baseline bone density test.[13] Then, in the future, your physician will compare the results of your baseline test to follow-up examinations to find out if you are losing bone. Check with your doctor to see which test he or she recommends. Many use photon energy to measure bone mass and predict possible fracture. Your doctor may also order blood and urine tests to look at bone metabolism.

An important prevention tip for women nearing menopause is to examine family history. If your mother and grandmother had signs of osteoporosis—if they lost

---

[13] Editorial, "Osteoporosis and Hip Fractures: Challenges to Investigators and Clinicians," Journal of the American Medical Association, February 2, 1990, p. 708.

height; broke their hips, spine, or wrist; lost their teeth; or had other significant symptoms—you should step up preventive measures. Finally, as you near menopause, record your height every year at least. If you start to lose height, get in touch with your doctor to evaluate you for osteoporosis.

<u>SUMMING UP</u>

Because we've covered so much ground—from bone remodeling to Type I and Type II osteoporosis—a quick summary will help review the major points covered in the previous pages.

- Osteoporosis is a disease that causes broken bones, resulting in pain, deformity, and disability.

- Osteoporosis is frighteningly common and increasingly striking at young ages.

- Osteoporosis is a silent disabler; it sneaks up on its victims and usually goes unnoticed until fractures occur.

- Osteoporosis develops when bone remodeling goes awry due to exposure to risk factors, such as decreasing estrogen levels, poor nutrition, or lack of weight-bearing exercise.

• The first principle of osteoporosis prevention is to build up a bone surplus during childhood and the early adult years.

• A second important principle is to maintain a strong bone structure during older age, when accumulated risk factors can result in osteoporosis.

• Women are highly vulnerable to developing osteoporosis. Estrogen replacement therapy is vital to prevent bone wasting after menopause.

• Happily, osteoporosis can be prevented and, if it occurs, treated, by adopting the steps described in the following chapters. <u>And, by adopting the steps to osteoporosis prevention, you will feel and look better. Your overall health and appearance will be youthful, and you will avoid the depression and isolation that often accompany osteoporosis.</u>

CHAPTER TWO

STEP ONE—LEARN THE RISK FACTORS FOR OSTEOPOROSIS

Osteoporosis is better prevented than treated. Since Galileo's time scientists have been examining how to prevent bone loss. A long tradition of research has led to a list of risk factors for osteoporosis that have been painstakingly identified. It is important to learn about these factors, described in this chapter, to identify if you are at high risk for osteoporosis and what you can do about it.

We have no control over some of these risk factors—being a woman, fair skinned, or slight of build, for example. These characteristics serve as warnings. If you have one or more of them you are likely to develop osteoporosis. In addition, the factors that are under our control are important for all of us. If you are a heavy smoker who can't break the habit, for example, you should be stepping up preventive measures for osteoporosis, because it is highly likely that your smoking habit is destroying your bones.

Finally, some health conditions and medications can lead to osteoporosis. If you have any of the conditions or are taking any of the medications listed in this chapter, you are at risk for developing osteoporosis.

The following provides a breakdown of the major risk factors for osteoporosis.[1]

THE FACTORS YOU CAN'T PREVENT

Being a Woman

Osteoporosis is six to eight times more common in women than in men. There are two major reasons for this: women have less bone mass to begin with, and, for several years after menopause, women lose bone rapidly when their body's production of estrogen declines.

Early Menopause

The National Institute of Health refers to an early menopause (before age 45) as a strong predictor for the

---

[1] Based on National Osteoporosis Foundation, "Stand Up to Osteoporosis," (Washington, D.C.: NOF, 1992); information provided by the National Institute of Arthritis, Musculoskeletal Diseases and Skin Diseases, (1993); and A. Paganini-Hill et al., "Exercise and Other Factors in the Prevention of Hig Fracture: The Leisure World Survey," Epidemiology, Vol. 2, no. 1, 1991, pp. 16-25.

development of osteoporosis. This is true whether the early menopause occurs naturally or is caused by surgical removal of the ovaries.

Fair Skin

Fair-skinned people are at greater risk than are those with dark skin. One explanation for this curious fact is that blacks naturally have higher rates of the bone-protecting hormone calcitonin. However, black American women should not be complacent. The percentage of African-American women with osteoporosis is increasing.[2]

Immobilization

Limited movement of specific body parts causes rapid loss of bone in the affected area. Patients confined to bed and astronauts under weightless conditions lose up to 1 percent of trabecular bone mass per week.[3] Happily,

---

[2] Carletta Joy Walker, "Healthy Bones," Essence, December 1992, p. 20.

[3] Sally S. Harris et al., "Physical Activity Counseling for Healthy Adults," Journal of the American Medical Association, June 23-30, 1989, p. 3592.

going back to weight-bearing exercise restores the bone to normal.

Being Thin and Small Boned

Women who are small boned and petite are at great risk for osteoporosis. Some researchers say that anyone weighing less than 140 pounds has a greater risk of osteoporosis.[4] This puts all women who are trying to reach the American ideal of slimness at great risk for developing osteoporosis.

Advancing Age

With each decade, the risk of hip fracture doubles.[5]

---

[4] Linda Ojeda, Menopause Without Medicine, (Alameda, CA: Hunter House, 1992), p. 57.

[5] Steven Cummings et al., "Appendicular Bone Density and Age Predict Hip Fracture in Women," Journal of the American Medical Association, February 2, 1990, p. 665.

A Family History of Osteoporosis

Anyone whose grandparents or parents have had signs of osteoporosis is at greater risk for developing the condition. For example, a recent study reported in the New England Journal of Medicine found that daughters of women with osteoporosis have weakened bone in the spine and hip.[6] According to Dr. David Fardon, author of Osteoporosis, "the highest incidence [of osteoporosis] is usually found among women whose mothers showed signs of osteoporosis."[7]

Medical Conditions

Many illnesses can cause bone thinning. They include chronic renal failure, Cushing's syndrome, Paget's disease, hyperparathyroidism, kidney disease, intestinal absorption disorders, liver disease, rheumatoid arthritis, diabetes, and certain cancers such as lymphoma and leukemia. Diabetics and people with hypogly-

---

[6] Ego Seeman et al., "Reduced Bone Mass in Daughters of Women with Osteoporosis," New England Journal of Medicine, March 2, 1989, p. 554.

[7] David F. Fardon, Osteoporosis, (New York: Macmillan, 1985), p. 15.

cemia can lose calcium when blood sugar levels are off balance. (See Chapter Three for more detail on these conditions.)

THE FACTORS YOU CAN PREVENT

A Diet Lacking in Calcium

Numerous studies have shown that lack of adequate calcium leads to osteoporosis. Calcium must be taken in daily to be effective. Unfortunately, <u>surveys have shown that most people do not consume as much calcium as they should to prevent bone loss</u>. For example, half of the women over age 44 consume less than half the amount of calcium they need per day.[8]

Lack of Weight-Bearing Exercise

A groundbreaking study of 14,000 men and women living in Leisure World, a retirement community in southern

---

[8] "For Older Women, Calcium Counts," <u>Newsweek</u>, October 8, 1990, p. 77.

California, found that lack of weight-bearing exercise leads to hip fracture.[9]

Too Much Exercise

For women, exercising to the point that monthly periods stop leads to osteoporosis. Several classic studies have been done in this area. In one study of 11 women runners in Boston who were not menstruating (amenorrhea), all 11 had significantly reduced bone density.

Smoking Cigarettes

In the Leisure World study mentioned earlier, cigarette smokers had a significantly increased risk of osteoporosis. In addition, there is evidence that the cadmium in cigarettes can lead to osteoporosis.[10]

---

[9] Paganini-Hill et al., "Exercise and Other Factors in the Prevention of Hip Fracture," pp. 16-25.

[10] "Cadmium May Speed Bone Loss in Women," Science News, December 3, 1988, p. 356.

Excessive Use of Alcohol

A 1991 report in the American Journal of Clinical Nutrition has shown that drinking even moderate amounts of alchohol daily doubles the likelihood of fracturing a hip.[11]

Prolonged Use of Specific Medications

Many medications can cause bone thinning. For example, excessive doses of thyroid medication, prescribed for low metabolism, lead to bone loss. Thyroid hormones are one of the most frequently prescribed drugs for women.[12] Other drugs that cause bone loss are the anticoagulant

---

[11] Mauricio Hernandez-Avila et al., "Caffeine, Moderate Alcohol Intake, and Risk Fractures of the Hip and Forearm in Middle-Aged Women," American Journal of Clinical Nutrition, Vol. 54, no. 1, pp. 157-63.

[12] Annie Kung and K. K. Pun, "Bone Mineral Density in Premenopausal Women Receiving Long-Term Physiological Doses of Levothyroxine," Journal of the American Medical Association, May 22, 1991, p. 2688.

heparin, antiseizure medications, certain diuretics, certain antibiotics, and corticosteroids. (See Chapter Three for more detail on these medications.)

Eating Disorders

Anorexia nervosa leads to weight loss, malnutrition, and loss of bone mass. Bone mass is not fully restored after return to normal weight.[13]

Regular Fasting and Strenuous Dieting

These activities result in bone wasting. For example, scientists at the Grand Forks Human Nutrition Research Center found that losing weight results in lost bone mass.[14] The ultrathin model may be enviable on the cover

---

[13] Nancy Rigotti et al., "The Clinical Course of Osteoporosis in Anorexia Nervosa," Journal of the American Medical Association, March 6, 1991, p. 1133.

[14] Jane Brody, "Health Pages," The New York Times, October 14, 1992, p. B7.

of Vogue, but imitating her could cause serious damage to bones.

High-Protein Intake

Many researchers have found that diets that are too high in protein cause loss of calcium and bone.[15] [16]

FACTORS THAT ARE SUSPICIOUS

These factors may lead to osteoporosis:

Over Consumption of Caffeine

Excessive caffeine consumption has long been suspected as a contributor to osteoporosis. Coffee, for example, is a diuretic, which causes loss of calcium in the urine. A recent study of over 84,000 American women ages 34 to

---

[15] Jane Brody, Jane Brody's Nutrition Book, (New York: W. W. Norton, 1981), p. 302.

[16] Jeffrey Bland, Nutraerobics, (New York: Harper & Row, 1983), p. 256.

59 found that high caffeine intake—primarily through drinking coffee—increases risk of hip, but not forearm, fracture. However, other studies have found only a weak link between caffeine and osteoporosis.[17]

Being Childless

According to one study, two-thirds of the women with osteoporosis are childless.[18]

Drinking Cola

For a long time, regular cola drinking has been suspected to lead to osteoporosis. However, in studies on rats, researchers at Mt. Sinai Hospital in Baltimore have found no connection between cola drinking and thinning bones.[19] Some skeptics are still suspicious of cola drinks, however, because of their high phosphorous content, which can block calcium absorption.

---

[17] Hernandez-Avila et al., "Caffeine, Moderate Alcohol Intake, and Risk Fractures of the Hip and Forearm in Middle-Aged Women," pp. 157-163.

[18] Ojeda, Menopause Without Medicine, p. 60.

[19] "Let Them Drink Cola," Science News, November 3, 1990, p. 286.

HEALTH CONDITIONS THAT LEAD TO OSTEOPOROSIS

Osteoporosis often occurs because of another medical problem. The following is a list of medical conditions that can lead to osteoporosis. If you have any of these problems, you should step up osteoporosis prevention measures:

Conditions Affecting Absorption
of Nutrients from Food

Types of conditions include bowel disease, intestinal problems, pancreas problems, or liver problems.

Kidney Disease and Kidney Stones

Both conditions may upset calcium excretion and absorption.

Amenorrhea

This condition occurs in women who stop menstruating. Research physiologist Barbara Drinkwater, at Pacific Medical Center, was one of the first to discover that women with amenorrhea resulting from overexercising develop weak bones. Drinkwater described the bones of five women with amenorrhea from a 1984 study of women who exercised too much. The five women reduced their exercise and started to menstruate again. The women, who are now in their thirties, have bones Drinkwater describes as "twenty years older."

Anorexia Nervosa

This is an eating disorder that results in malnutrition. In one study, using a diagnostic procedure called dual photon absorptiometry, two-thirds of the young adolescent women with anorexia had significant bone loss.[20]

Any Condition That Reduces Estrogen Levels

If the condition continues long enough, it results in osteoporosis. Conditions that reduce or shut off estrogen include loss of the ovaries, lack of periods (amenorrhea), and menopause.

Elevated Levels of the Hormone Prolactin

This hormone is responsible for stimulating milk production after childbirth.

Excess Thyroid

This condition, called hyperthyroidism, can disturb the balance of calcium and phosphorous.

----

[20] Iris F. Litt, "Adolescent Medicine," Journal of the American Medical Association, June 19, 1991, p. 3101.

Diabetes

This disorder of carbohydrate metabolism can cause excess bone loss and decreased bone formation.

Lactase Deficiency

The inability to digest milk often results in avoidance of dairy products, which then leads to osteoporosis.

Any Condition Causing Immobilization

Conditions such as polio, paralysis, spondylitis, lung conditions, Parkinson's disease, and arthritis can lead to osteoporosis.

Cushing's Syndrome

This is a condition caused by overproduction of glucocorticoids by the adrenal glands, which leads to osteoporosis.

Alcoholism

Excessive drinking results in osteoporosis through many effects, including decreasing estrogen levels, reducing bone construction (through directly modifying osteoblast activity), and poor nutrition. Alcoholics are also at greater jeopardy for falling and fracturing bones.

Surgery for Obesity

Types of surgery include stapling the stomach or gastric bypass. Such surgery can seriously upset calcium absorption.

Surgical Removal of the Stomach

Calcium absorption is dramatically upset.

MEDICATIONS THAT LEAD TO OSTEOPOROSIS

Excessive use of certain medications can also lead to osteoporosis. They include the following:

Corticosteroids

Regular or excessive use of steroids, used to treat asthma, arthritis, allergic reactions, cancer, and other medical conditions, leads to serious bone thinning. Corticosteroids include cortisone and prednisone. Fortunately, inhalation of steroids does not cause the same problem. Steroids should be taken for the shortest amount of time possible.

Anticonvulsants

These drugs include phenytoin (Dilantin™) and phenobarbital, which can cause vitamin D deficiencies and hamper calcium absorption.

Aluminum-Containing Antacids

Popular remedies include Alka-Seltzer™ and Digel™, which can cause calcium excretion.

Diuretics Made with Furosemide

These diuretics increase loss of calcium. Stick to thiazide diuretics, which reduce calcium excretion.

Thyroid Medication

Treatment for hypothyroidism can cause too much bone demolition during remodeling.[21]

Heparin

A blood thinner, this drug leads to osteoporosis.

Tetracycline

This antibiotic interferes with bone growth.

---

[21] Felicia Stewart, Felicia Guest, Gary Stewart, and Robert Hatcher, Understanding Your Body, (New York: Bantam, 1987), p. 598.

CHAPTER THREE

STEP TWO—DEVELOP A WELL-ROUNDED,

HIGH-CALCIUM NUTRITION PROGRAM

Step two of osteoporosis prevention is to develop a well-rounded, high-calcium nutrition program. This chapter covers basic information on the low-calcium/osteoporosis link and provides tips on how to make sure that you take in enough calcium. (High-calcium recipes are included in the appendix to this report.)

CALCIUM

Like brushing your teeth and feeding the family cat, consuming adequate calcium should be an important part of your daily routine. Not only your bones, but every cell in your body, requires calcium to function.

Calcium is the most plentiful mineral in your body. If it were not present, your muscles would not contract and your brain would shut down. Even your blood depends on calcium and, without it, cannot clot. The evidence is clear. Without calcium, we would be like fish out of water.

Calcium is not only crucial to human beings, but it is also an essential component of the earth and its creatures. It is found in rocks, soil, and all bodies of water. It is in all animals and plants, in seashells, eggshells, and marble.

Many studies have shown that lack of adequate calcium leads to osteoporosis. According to the National Osteoporosis Foundation, lack of calcium during childhood can cause as much as a 5 to 7 percent difference in peak bone mass.[1] Recently, New Zealand researchers found calcium supplements of 1,000 milligrams (mg) per day reduce bone loss in women who are at least three years past menopause by one-half to one-third.[2]

Calcium deficiency can cause other health problems, including periodontal disease, which is the breakdown of the bones supporting the teeth. The condition is the

---

[1] National Osteoporosis Foundation, Physician's Resource Manual on Osteoporosis, 2nd ed. (Washington, D.C.: NOF, 1991) p. 21.

[2] Ian R. Reid, "The Effect of Calcium Supplementation on Bone Loss in Postmenopausal Women," New England Journal of Medicine, February 18, 1993, pp. 460-464.

top cause of tooth loss in the United States today. Lack of calcium also causes high blood pressure, which can lead to strokes, heart attacks, and kidney disease. It also causes the soft bones and bowed legs of rickets in children.

Calcium and Development of the Skeleton

Different stages of life cause different demands for calcium. During childhood and early adulthood when bones are developing their length and strength, the most important nutrients are protein and energy-producing foods. Calcium plays an essential, but secondary, role. However, even during this stage, children, particularly girls, often do not get the calcium they need for optimum bone development. Girls age 10 to 11 consume on the average 55 to 60 percent of the calcium they require.[3] This means their bones will never reach peak bone mass and their risk of developing osteoporosis is very high.

---

[3] J. J. B. Anderson and R. C. Henderson, "Dietary Factor in the Development of Peak Bone Mass," in Nutritional Aspects of Osteoporosis, Serona Symposia, Vol. 85 (New York: Raven Press, 1991), p. 4.

For women, pregnancy, nursing, and the postmenopause years are also important. During pregnancy and nursing, the baby's needs are met at the expense of the mother's bones, unless calcium intake is increased. At least a 50 percent increase in calcium intake is recommended during pregnancy.[4] (This recommendation is discussed later in this chapter.) In addition, the loss of estrogen that occurs with menopause causes a sharp increase in the rate of bone resorption. Need for calcium also increases during this time.

As mentioned in Chapter One, under normal circumstances nerves, muscles, and other parts of the body receive calcium from the bloodstream. However, if there is not enough of the nutrient available through this source, your body uses bone as backup reserves, drawing the nutrient out of your skeleton, into your blood. This process gradually weakens bones, leaving them starved for calcium.

Unfortunately, it may be decades before an individual realizes that he or she has calcium deficiency. At this

---

[4] Jane Brody, Jane Brody's Nutrition Book, (New York: W. W. Norton, 1981), p. 335.

point it is too late to prevent the pain and creeping disability of repeated fractures. This is why building up a little extra bone, which acts like an auxiliary calcium supply, is so important to prevent osteoporosis.

Calcium must be taken daily to replace the calcium lost through elimination and perspiration. Unfortunately, surveys have shown most people do not consume as much calcium as they should to replace the loss. For example, half of the women over age 44 consume less than half the amount of calcium they need per day.[5] And the typical American diet provides about 300 mg of calcium per day, one-fifth the recommended amount for many.[6]

Calcium Absorption

Many factors cause poor absorption of calcium. It is absorbed less efficiently with increasing age, for

---

[5] "For Older Women, Calcium Counts," Newsweek, October 8, 1990, p. 77.

[6] Bess Dawson-Hughes et al., "A Controlled Trial of the Effect of Calcium Supplementation on Bone Density in Postmenopausal Women," New England Journal of Medicine, Vol. 323, no. 13, September 27, 1990, p. 624.

example. The following factors also may decrease your body's ability to absorb calcium:

- Disease or illness

- Lack of estrogen

- Lack of exercise

- Certain medications

- Smoking

- Caffeine

- Stress

- Lack of important vitamins and minerals such as vitamin D and magnesium

- An inherited inability to absorb calcium efficiently

Daily Calcium Guidelines

The best source of calcium is food. Many foods are rich in the nutrient, including milk, yogurt, cheese, other dairy products, and canned salmon. Even green leafy vegetables are a good source of calcium. In fact, cows get all the calcium they need from eating grass. Happily, even so-called "junk foods" such as Pizza Hut's supreme personal pan pizza and macaroni and cheese can be great sources of calcium. (For a detailed list of calcium-rich foods and fast-food sources of calcium, see Table 3-1 beginning on page 62 of this chapter.)

To make sure your diet contains adequate calcium, include a dairy product at every meal. Calcium is absorbed more efficiently when taken throughout the day. The National Osteoporosis Foundation suggests never taking more than 500 or 600 mg of calcium at a time. According to the foundation, "Smaller doses several times a day are more easily absorbed by the body."

At each meal drink a glass of skim milk; or grate low-fat cheese over your salad or soup; or eat canned salmon (with bones), frozen yogurt, or broccoli with melted cheese. (Leave the leaves on the broccoli when you cook it, because they contain most of the calcium.) Many experts recommend taking calcium at night so it does not have to compete with anything else for absorption. Milk is calming. Drinking a glass before you go to bed may help you fall asleep.

Sadly, human beings are the only animals who do not get adequate calcium. A common explanation for this is the average diet of humans, which is high in fat and protein, neither of which contain the nutrient. The best calcium intake guidelines were developed in 1984 by a conference sponsored by the National Institutes of Health, called the Consensus Development Conference on Osteoporosis. The top osteoporosis experts in the country attended the conference to reach consensus on how to prevent and treat osteoporosis.

The panel found that premenopausal and older women receiving estrogen need about 1,000 mg of elemental calcium per day to keep the amount of calcium in the bones constant. Women past the age of menopause who are not on estrogen need about 1,500 mg of elemental calcium per day (to prevent Type I and II bone loss). In addition, adult men should take in 1,000 mg of elemental calcium to prevent age-related (Type II) bone loss.

As mentioned earlier, children must take in adequate calcium to build as much bone mass as possible. A recent study at Indiana University found increasing the calcium intake of children creates higher bone density than average intake. (Researchers compared intakes of 1,612 mg versus 908 mg per day.)

The recommended guidelines for children are[7]

Age	Milligrams of Elemental Calcium per Day
Birth-0.5 years	360
0.5-1	540
1-10	800
10-18	1,200

A word of warning: The old adage that you can get too much of a good thing holds true for calcium. Taking in over 2,500 mg of calcium per day may cause absorption problems for other important minerals such as iron or zinc. Taking too much calcium can also cause kidney or gall bladder stones in people who are susceptible to them.

You're Never Too Old

Whatever your age, adding calcium to your diet can restore some bone mass. Researchers at Tufts University in Massachusetts found calcium makes a big difference for women whose menopause occurred more than five years previously, including those who are elderly. In this group, women who ate less than 400 mg of calcium daily

---

[7] Data are from National Academy of Sciences, National Research Council.

still had significant bone loss in the hip, spine, and forearm. However, increasing their calcium intake to just 800 mg daily decreased their bone loss significantly.[8] This finding did not hold true for women who were within five years of the end of their periods. For these women, only estrogen replacement stopped bone loss.

If You Are Pregnant or Nursing

To protect your bone density, and your baby's, it is important to take in additional calcium when pregnant or nursing. Here are some guidelines from the Osteoporosis Foundation:

Pregnant or Nursing	Milligrams of Elemental Calcium per Day
Under 19 years old	1,600
19 years or older	1,200

Calcium Supplements

Calcium supplements can play an important role in the prevention of osteoporosis, but choosing the right one

---

[8] Dawson-Hughes et al., "A Controlled Trial of the Effect of Calcium Supplementation on Bone Density in Postmenopausal Women," p. 878.

can be confusing, because not all forms are alike.
Moreover, when taking supplements, it is easy to get too
much.

To find out if a supplement will meet your daily
requirements, count the amount of <u>elemental calcium</u> each
supplement contains. <u>Elemental calcium is the type of</u>
<u>calcium your body can use.</u> Different forms of calcium
contain different amounts of elemental calcium. For
example, 100 mg of calcium carbonate contain 40 mg of
elemental calcium and 250 mg of calcium lactate contain
34 mg of elemental calcium.

A terrific source of elemental calcium is the antacid
Tums-EX™. Each tablet contains 300 mg of elemental
calcium. Postmenopausal women on estrogen supplementation should take four tablets a day (1,200 mg of elemental
calcium). Postmenopausal women not on estrogen should
take five tablets (1,500 mg). <u>However, watch out for</u>
<u>other calcium-containing antacids that also contain</u>
<u>aluminum.</u> They can block the absorption of calcium and
lead to other problems.

Supplements that contain calcium carbonate may cause
constipation, nausea, or gas. Drinking lots of water and
including plenty of fiber in the diet may cut down on

these effects. However, this is a Catch 22, because taking calcium with a high-fiber meal also can reduce calcium absorption.

When selecting a calcium supplement, stick to those meeting United States Pharmacopeia (USP) standards, which guarantee that they can be absorbed. Some supplements, including those sold in health food stores, are not easily absorbed. Your druggist can tell you which supplements meet USP standards. Avoid dolomite and bone meal products, which your local health food store may feature as a calcium supplement. Both contain lead.

If you have a calcium supplement on your vitamin shelf you are not sure about, try the "vinegar test." Put a tablet in a glass of vinegar and stir occasionally. Three quarters of the supplement will dissolve in half an hour if the supplement is <u>bioavailable,</u> which means your body can absorb it.

What Are USRDAs?

Many people have questions about US Recommended Dietary Allowances (USRDAs), which are listed on most food labels. USRDAs are suggested levels of nutrient intakes and labeling standards set by scientists at the U.S.

Food and Drug Administration (FDA). The USRDA for calcium is 1,000 mg per day.

USRDAs are often expressed as percentages. This represents the percentage of the daily recommendation for calcium a particular product fills. For example, if the label on a box of powdered dry milk says 5 tablespoons contains 30 percent USRDA of calcium, then this amount equals 300 mg of calcium.

Most experts on osteoporosis do not agree with the USRDAs but advise adults and postmenopausal women to take in higher levels of calcium.[9] Their recommendations are based on many studies that show that boosting calcium intake beyond the USRDAS significantly increases bone density. In other words, it is important to understand that USRDAs are too low for most individuals.

Examples of Calcium Intake

It is hard to keep track of how much calcium you take in every day. Here are some examples of how to make sure you get at least 1,000 mg of calcium a day:

---

[9] Includes findings from conferences sponsored in 1987 and 1990 by the National Institutes of Health and the National Osteoporosis Foundation.

- 2 glasses of skim milk, 3 ounces of salmon, 1 ounce of Swiss cheese

    Breakfast—Cereal with a cup of milk

    Lunch—Sandwich with 1 ounce of Swiss cheese

    Dinner—3 ounces of salmon

    Bedtime snack—1 glass of skim milk

- 1 cup plain low-fat yogurt, 1 ounce American cheese, 2 spears broccoli, 1 tablespoon molasses in a cup of skim milk

    Breakfast—1 cup plain yogurt with fruit

    Dinner—2 steamed broccoli spears with 1 ounce of American cheese melted on top

    Late-night snack—1 glass of heated milk with a tablespoon of molasses, cinnamon, and nutmeg added to it

If You Have Trouble Digesting Milk

If drinking milk causes digestion problems, you may lack the enzyme lactase, which aids digestion of a milk sugar called lactose. However, you can eat other dairy products, such as yogurt and buttermilk made from cultured milk, hard cheeses, and acidophilus milk, in which the lactose has been broken down. Natural cheeses contain only small amounts of lactose. Fermented cheeses have the least. You can also treat dairy products with lactase drops or take lactase pills to facilitate digesting lactose. Both may be found in most drug-stores.

The Fat Problem

When confronted with adding calcium to your diet, you may feel discouraged by the amount of fat and calories found in many dairy products. You may think, "I'll put on weight and put myself at risk for getting heart disease." However, there are many ways to get adequate calcium and still keep calories and fat counts way down. For example, skim milk has an average of 90 calories per cup, compared to about 150 for whole milk.

A quick rule of thumb is most hard cheeses are loaded with calcium but are also heavy in fat and calories. However, many excellent low-fat or nonfat cheeses are now on the market. Most do not sacrifice calcium. Cottage cheese, part-skim ricotta, and nonfat yogurt are excellent sources of calcium, for example.

<u>Foods and Nutrients That Affect</u>
<u>Calcium Absorption</u>

Different foods may block calcium absorption, cause it
to be excreted, or enhance its absorption.[10] Obviously,
you should emphasize the enhancers in your diet and
de-emphasize the excreters. Two elements often mentioned
are magnesium and zinc. Too much magnesium can prevent
bone calcification, and too little can impede bone
development. However, a balanced diet provides all the
magnesium that is needed; deficiency is extremely rare.
Zinc aids bone calcification. The USRDA is 15 milligrams.
Many experts think that drinking coffee and other
caffeine-containing products, smoking cigarettes, and
taking in too much protein and sodium cause calcium to
be excreted from the body. Other culprits include
antacids with aluminum, phosphorous in soft drinks and

---

[10] This section is adapted from the National Osteoporosis
Foundation, <u>Boning Up on Osteoporosis</u>, (Washington,
D.C.: NOF, 1991) pp. 22-23.

protein-rich foods, and ecolates in tea. Extreme amounts
of fiber, found in fruits, vegetables, whole grain bread,
cereal products, and bran, also interfere with calcium
absorption.[11] On the other hand, both vitamin D and
lactose enhance calcium absorption.

Some foods that are rich in calcium also contain a
substance called oxalic acid, which can hinder calcium
absorption. Oxalic acid is found in spinach, kale,
mustard greens, rhubarb, and chocolate.[12]

Phosphorous is key to efficient calcium absorption,
but on average Americans get too much of this nutrient,
not too little. Phosphorous is present in red meat,

---

[11] For individuals on diets that contain high amounts of
insoluble fiber, foods with oxalates and phytates
should be avoided. Oxalates and phytates combine with
calcium in the intestines, and together they cannot
be absorbed. Foods that contain oxalates include
spinach, beets, parsley, rhubarb, summer squash,
peanuts, tea, and cocoa. Products that contain
phytates include legumes and, possibly, wheat bran.

[12] Joanne Ness and Genell Subak-Sharpe, The Calcium
Requirement Cookbook, (New York: M. Evans, 1985), p.
13.

processed foods such as luncheon meats and cheeses, white bread, soft drinks, and packaged pastries. Most of these should be eliminated from your diet. You also should restrict all foods containing the following: potassium phosphate, sodium phosphate, phosphoric acid, pyrophosphate, or polyphosphate.

Adding Calcium to Your Diet

Here are some tips for adding calcium to your diet:

- Drink skim milk with meals or as a snack. Skim milk has slightly more calcium than whole milk and is greatly reduced in fat.

- Use reduced-fat milk or nonfat dry milk to prepare foods such as casseroles, soups, sauces, and beverages. Add a couple of tablespoons of powdered milk to casseroles to boost the calcium content.

- Add nonfat dried milk to juices or buy calcium-fortified orange, grapefruit, or apple juice.

- Preserve nutrients in vegetables high in calcium by cooking them in a steamer or a very small amount of water for a very short time.

- Eat canned salmon, tuna, and sardines including the bones, which are rich in calcium.

- Replace cream with evaporated skim milk. Evaporated skim milk is creamy and works well in gravies, soups, and sauces.

- Use dry milk or evaporated skim milk as coffee creamer.

- Buy products with "nonfat milk solids" added. They significantly boost calcium content.

- Make low-fat yogurt cheese with a coffee filter or a cone, sold in health food stores for this purpose. It is a wonderful substitute for cream cheese. Eat it on toast with sugar-free jam or stir into soup or curry. Not only is the cheese high in calcium, but the whey, which is the watery liquid that drips out of the filter or cone, is chock full of calcium and other water-soluble vitamins. Yogurt whey can be added to other foods such as soups, breads, and drinks to boost their vitamin content. The Swiss drink sweetened whey as a soft drink.[13]

---

[13] Sharon Stocker, "Short and Sweet," Prevention, January 1993, p. 144.

Milk Products

There are many types of milk products from which to choose, all of which are storehouses of calcium. Because they differ by the amount of fat they contain, choosing the right dairy product can be confusing for the diet conscious. One important point to remember is that milk products with reduced fat are as nutritious as whole milk. Sometimes, they are more nutritious. Here is a breakdown of milk products and the amount of fat they provide. All are full of calcium.

Whole milk contains at least 3.25 percent fat and 8.25 percent other nonfat "solids" providing protein and carbohydrates. Every quart must contain at least 2,000 I.U. (international units) of vitamin A and 400 I.U. of vitamin D.

Low-fat milk has from 0.5 to 2 percent fat and, like whole milk, at least 8.25 percent nonfat solids. Often different types of low-fat milk will use their percentage fat as their name such as "1% milk" or "2% milk."

Skim or nonfat milk has less than .5 percent fat.

Buttermilk is reduced-fat milk with a tart flavor. A culture is added to the milk to ferment the milk sugar.

Contrary to what its name suggests, it does not contain butter and is low in fat.

Yogurt, like buttermilk, is the result of adding a culture to milk. Yogurt made from whole milk has at least 3.25 percent fat. When made from low-fat milk, it has 0.5 percent to 2 percent fat. When made from nonfat milk it has less than 0.5 percent milk.

Sour cream is also made from milk and a culture. It contains 18 percent fat.

Cream contains not less than 18 percent fat. However, fat levels for different types of cream range from 10.5 percent fat (some brands of half-and-half cream) to 36 percent fat (heavy cream).

Nonfat dry milk can be kept on the pantry shelf for a very long time without spoiling. It is nutritionally the same as other types of milk.

Evaporated milk is whole or nonfat milk that has had over half the water removed.

For a breakdown of the amount of calcium in each of these dairy products see Table 3-1.

Calcium Is Not the Bottom Line

It is important to remember that adequate calcium is important to preventing osteoporosis, but it is not a replacement for hormone therapy for women and exercise for both women and men. In other words, effectively thwarting the disease means practicing all the osteoporosis prevention steps together.

VITAMIN D

The sun vitamin, vitamin D, plays a critical role in osteoporosis prevention. Vitamin D is produced in the skin through exposure to sunlight or is found in dairy products. The body must have the vitamin available to absorb calcium efficiently. If you do not get enough of the vitamin, your diet should be extremely high in calcium to compensate for the insufficiency. Up to 60 percent of individuals who fracture a hip may have vitamin D deficiency.[14] You should be taking in about 400 I.U. of the vitamin daily.

Unlike calcium, vitamin D is not readily available in the diets of most animals, including human beings. The usual way of taking it in is from the sun's rays. Vitamin

---

[14] Marie C. Chapuy et al., "Vitamin D3 and Calcium to Prevent Fractures in Elderly Women," New England Journal of Medicine, Vol. 327, no. 23, 1992, p. 1637.

D is formed in the body when ultraviolet light interacts with cholesterol molecules in the body. In humans this interaction occurs in the middle of the skin; in other animals it occurs on their fur or feathers. Vitamin D is stored in body fat, where the body can build up reserves for rainy days.

Most experts say 15 minutes a day of sun exposure provides enough vitamin D to meet the body's requirements. If you are outdoors every day for about 30 minutes, you do not need to take vitamin D supplements.[15] (You have to be outdoors to take in ultraviolet light; it does not go through glass.) If you do not get much sun or eat or drink many dairy products, you should take a supplement. Use caution, however, like calcium, too much of the "sun" vitamin can cause problems. Toxicity can occur at levels as low as 2,000 I.U. daily and can lead to kidney stones and high blood levels of calcium. The National Osteoporosis Foundation recommends not taking more than 1,000 I.U. of vitamin D daily.

---

[15] Karyn Holm and Jane Walker, _Geriatric Nursing_, May-June 1990, pp. 141-142.

Vitamin D deficiency is a problem for anyone who lives in an institution or is homebound. In fact, an adult form of rickets resulting from lack of vitamin D is common among elderly persons with fractures.

FAT, PROTEIN, AND SUGAR

Bone diseases are found in societies where high levels of protein are consumed and are rare where the diet is primarily vegetarian. Many researchers have found diets that are too high in protein cause loss of calcium and bone, while vegetarian diets help to ward off osteoporosis.[16] [17] Studies also have shown vegetarians lose less bone than meat eaters with age.[18]

---

[16] Brody, Jane Brody's Nutrition Book, p. 302.

[17] Jeffrey Bland, Nutraerobics (New York: Harper & Row, 1983), p. 256.

[18] Robin Marantz Henig, How a Woman Ages, (Cambridge, Mass.: Ballantine, 1985), p. 81.

Doubling protein consumption causes a 50 percent increase in calcium loss.[19] One explanation is that meat and poultry, major sources of protein in the diet, are low in calcium. They also have a number of characteristics that block calcium absorption or cause its excretion by the kidneys, including high phosphorous content.

To cut down on protein, you can substitute pasta, grains, beans, vegetables, and fruits.

Fat consumption that is too high or too low also affects efficient calcium absorption. However, calcium requires the presence of some fat for efficient use by the body. Even M and Ms and Reese's Pieces are troublemakers where calcium is concerned. Too much sugar causes stomach acidity that results in excretion of calcium from the bones.

SUMMING UP

Here is a quick summary of the basics in step two:

---

[19] Frederick S. Kaplan, Osteoporosis, Health Needs of Women as They Age, (New York: Haworth Press, 1985), p. 97.

- Take in adequate calcium, preferably through your diet. If your diet is inadequate in calcium, take a daily supplement. Use the guidelines in this chapter to establish how much calcium you and your family need during different periods of life.

- Get fifteen minutes a day of sun exposure or take a vitamin D supplement. But do not take more than 1000 I.U. of vitamin D daily.

- Limit your fat and protein intake. Also, cut down on other foods that block calcium absorption.

Table 3-1
Some Calcium-Rich Foods

	Measure	Calories	Calcium Available (mg)
Dairy			
Cheese			
Blue	1 ounce	100	150
Cheddar	1 ounce	115	204
Feta	1 ounce	75	140
Mozzarella, whole milk	1 ounce	80	147
Mozzarella, skim milk	1 ounce	80	207

	Measure	Calories	Calcium Available (mg)
Muenster	1 ounce	105	203
Parmesan, grated	1 tbsp	25	69
Pasteurized Process			
American	1 ounce	105	174
Swiss	1 ounce	95	219
Provolone	1 ounce	100	214
Swiss	1 ounce	105	272
Cottage Cheese			
Lowfat (2%)	1 cup	205	155
Creamed (4%)			
Large curd	1 cup	235	135
Small curd	1 cup	215	126
Milk			
Skim	1 cup	85	302
1% fat	1 cup	100	300
2% fat	1 cup	120	297
Whole	1 cup	150	291
Buttermilk	1 cup	100	285
Dry, nonfat, instant	¼ cup	61	209
Yogurt			
Plain, low-fat with added milk solids	1 cup	145	415

	Measure	Calories	Calcium Available (mg)
Fruit, low-fat with added milk solids	1 cup	230*	345*
Plain, whole milk	1 cup	140	274
Desserts			
Vanilla ice cream, hard, 11% fat	1 cup	270	176
Vanilla ice milk, hard 4% fat	1 cup	185	176
Vanilla ice milk, soft, 3% fat	1 cup	225	274
Seafood			
Oysters, raw	1 cup	160	226
Salmon, pink, canned, with bones	3 ounces	120	167
Sardines, canned, drained	3 ounces	175	371
Vegetables			
Bok choy, raw	1 cup	9	74
Broccoli, raw	1 spear	40	72
Collard greens, cooked	1 cup	60	357
Dandelion greens, cooked	1 cup	35	147
Kale, cooked	1 cup	40	179

	Measure	Calories	Calcium Available (mg)
Mustard greens, cooked	1 cup	20	104
Turnip greens, cooked	1 cup	50	249

Dried Beans

<u>Cooked, drained</u>

Great Northern	1 cup	210	90
Navy	1 cup	225	95
Pinto	1 cup	265	86
Chickpeas	1 cup	270	80
Soybeans	1 cup	235	131

<u>Canned</u>

Red kidney	1 cup	230	74
Refried beans	1 cup	295	141

Miscellaneous

Molasses, cane blackstrap	2 tbsp	85	274
Tofu	4 ounces	85	108–300†

* Values may vary.

† Tofu processed with calcium salts can have up to 300 mg calcium for a 4-ounce serving.

Calcium-Rich Foods/Fast Foods*

While the following foods are <u>not</u> recommended as a regular part of the diet, realistically there are times, for all of us, when fast foods are the only option. This list is included here to guide your food choice during those times.

Food	Calcium (mg)
Pizza Hut	
Supreme personal pan pizza	520
Lasagna (2½" × 2½")	460
Macaroni and cheese, 1 cup	362
Cheese enchilada	324
McDonald's	
Big Mac	256
Egg McMuffin	256
Filet-o-Fish	165
Wendy's	
Broccoli and cheese potato	250
Chef's salad without	235
dressing	224
Quiche (one-eighth pie)	224
Regular cheeseburger	182
Tomato soup with milk, 1 cup	159
Spaghetti and meat balls, 1 cup	124
Taco Bell's taco	84
Dairy Queen hot dog	80

* From <u>The All American Guide to Calcium Rich Foods</u>.
Courtesy of National Dairy Council®.

CHAPTER FOUR

STEP THREE—GET PLENTY OF WEIGHT-BEARING EXERCISE

Bones are like waistlines; they change according to the amount and type of exercise they get. In fact, your bones may change many times during your lifetime. Consider the following story of a woman who is now in her eighties:

During childhood Jean's bones grew tall and strong due to a sound diet with lots of calcium and daily exercise. By her early twenties, Jean's skeleton was strong and sturdy. Then she spent the next couple of decades working at a desk, drinking coffee, smoking, drinking a little alcohol during the week, and drinking a lot of alcohol on weekends. During this time, she delivered and nursed two children and did not take in adequate calcium. Jean's bones began to waste away for lack of exercise and poor nutrition.

At 40 Jean had a bad fall that fractured her wrist. After her doctor warned her that she was developing weak bones, she took up exercise with a vengeance. She played tennis 4 times a week for the next ten years and her right forearm grew thicker. She also quit smoking and cut down on her drinking. She walked four miles every other day. Jean's entire skeleton developed strength over the next decade.

Menopause struck in Jean's early fifties and because, at that time, estrogen was associated with cancer, she did not take hormone replacement therapy. Because she felt lousy, she also stopped exercising. Jean's bones began to waste away again. By 60 she had lost two inches in height, and she was in constant pain from spinal fractures. Now exercise was really out of the question.

Finally, at age 69, Jean started taking hormones, along with a daily calcium supplement. She also joined a water aerobics class for seniors and walks every day. Jean's bones will never be as strong as they could have been, but now she is reversing some of the thinning. She has not had any fractures since turning 70.

Jean's story points out the importance of maintaining step three of osteoporosis prevention: getting enough of the right kind of exercise, or "shaking those bones" as one osteoporosis expert calls it. One of Jean's problems was lack of weight-bearing exercise during the years when she worked at a desk.

What is weight-bearing exercise? It is exercise that places your bones against weight, gravity, or pressure. For example, walking and dancing are weight bearing, while bicycling and swimming are not. In short, exercise that is weight bearing increases bone mass. Not getting enough weight-bearing exercise decreases bone mass.

The connection between exercise and the size, shape, and strength of the skeletal system has been known at least since the seventeenth century. One of the best illustrations is what happened to the bodies of two Russian cosmonauts who spent 211 days in weightless space. They lost so much bone and muscle strength they could not walk for a week when they came back to earth.

Many other examples point out the importance of weight-bearing exercise. People who are immobilized develop osteoporosis in the affected bones. For example, people paralyzed by spinal cord injury lose one-third of the soft inner portion of their bones within six months of the injury.[1]

―――――――――――――

[1] David F. Fardon, <u>Osteoporosis</u>, (New York: Macmillan, 1985), p. 221.

While immobilization causes bone loss, people who use certain body parts over and over again build up bone density in that area. The shoulders of baseball pitchers, the legs of ballet dancers and long-distance runners, and the forearms of tennis players all illustrate this point.

Here is one woman's story of how exercise reversed her osteoporosis.

At age 50 Nora, like her mother 20 years before her, broke several vertebrae in her lower back. (Nora's mother is now age 87 and totally bedridden in a nursing home.)

After the fracture, Nora went on a serious exercise regimen, walking at least 2 miles a day and using a rowing machine every other day. While her mother was steadily losing bone when she was this age, a recent test shows that Nora's bone density increased by 1 percent over the last year.

Exercise not only builds strong bones. It also strengthens the heart and lungs, lowers blood pressure, stimulates circulation, and protects against adult-onset diabetes. It strengthens and tones muscle and keeps joints, tendons, and ligaments more flexible, all of which protect bones from fractures. Exercise also provides better bowel elimination and cuts down on the need for medications such as laxatives, sleeping pills, and pain killers. And there is more good news. If you exercise on a regular basis, you will have more energy, sleep better, and feel less tense. It will also be easier to control your weight and improve your appearance.

In short, exercise should be a lifelong project to build up peak bone mass and cut down on the natural bone loss that occurs with age. Even when begun later in life, exercise can reverse bone loss. The National Institutes on Health recommend at least three to four hours a week of weight-bearing exercise, such as brisk walking, running, tennis, or aerobic dance to prevent osteoporosis.

There are a number of weight-bearing exercises from which to choose, including walking, jogging, hiking, aerobic dancing, stair climbing, water walking, treadmill exercises, weight training, and jump roping. It is important to pick an exercise you will like so that you will stick to it. (But golf does not count as exercise, particularly if you ride in a cart.)

TYPES OF EXERCISE

There are two major types of exercise with differing weight-bearing benefits. <u>Aerobic</u> or <u>isotonic exercise</u> increases the heart rate while large muscles groups move for a long period of time. Most aerobic exercise is also weight bearing and bone strengthening. In other words, it places your bones against weight, gravity, or pressure. <u>Isometric exercise</u> does not increase the heart rate, but it does increase muscle strength. Examples are push-ups and weight lifting. Moderate amounts of isometric exercise are good for muscle strengthening and conditioning.

WALKING

Walking is one of the best weight-bearing exercises available for strengthening bones. It has the advantage of being free (except for the price of an excellent walking shoe, which is important to protect your bones). Walking strengthens bones as well as back and stomach muscles.

HOW TO START

The National Institutes of Health recommend beginning exercise slowly, especially if you are out of shape. Start with short periods. Then build up slowly, adding no more than a few minutes each week. If all goes well, slowly increase your exercise periods to 15 to 30 minutes, three or four times a week. It's also a good idea to include warm-up and cool-down periods of 5 to 15 minutes to tune up your body before exercise and to help wind down afterward. This should include stretching and then doing the same activity, but at a slower pace.

BE CAUTIOUS

The old saying that there can be too much of a good thing holds true for exercise. While not enough exercise results in bone loss, too much exercise also causes bone loss. This is particularly true for women who have poor diets and exercise so much they stop menstruating (a condition called amenorrhea).

If you are an athlete who is exercising to the point of not menstruating, you should cut back on exercising to ward off bone loss and consider one of three treatments: taking cyclic estrogen-progestin therapy, taking oral contraceptives, or inducing ovulation.[2] You

---

[2] Mona Shangold et al., "Evaluation and Management of Menstrual Dysfunction in Athletes," Journal of the American Medical Association, Vol. 263, no. 12, March 23-30, 1990, p. 1667.

should discuss these options with a well-informed physician.

Men also risk weakening their bones when they over-exercise and eat poorly. In men, prolonged overexercising coupled with a poor diet significantly reduces levels of the male hormone testosterone.

Strenuous exercise can be harmful. Pay attention to what your body tells you. If you have osteoporosis, or any other health condition, you should check with your doctor before doing any type of exercise. For example, if you have osteoporosis, you risk fracturing a bone. If you feel discomfort while exercising, you are trying to do too much. Be alert to the following: chest pain, breathlessness, joint discomfort, or muscle cramps. If you have any of these problems, call your doctor. However, the final analysis is that, for most of us, not exercising has far greater negative consequences than does exercising.

EXERCISE IS NOT THE BOTTOM LINE

While exercise is vitally important to prevent osteopo-rosis, it is not the bottom line. Barbara L. Drinkwater, a research physiologist and expert on osteoporosis, refers to women who exercise in place of taking estrogen to prevent osteoporosis as "playing Russian roulette with their bones."[3] Drinkwater points to the weakened bones of female athletes who exercise too much and lose their estrogen production as evidence that exercise without estrogen results in bone loss, not gain. And researchers have found that if exercise alone is the sole preventive measure used against osteoporosis, postmenopausal women would have to walk briskly two hours a day every day (or the equivalent) to halt bone loss.[4]

EXERCISES RECOMMENDED

BY THE NATIONAL OSTEOPOROSIS FOUNDATION

The following posture tips and exercises on pages 76-83 have been recommended by the National Osteoporosis Foundation.

---

[3] Comments made at the Second International Research Advances in Osteoporosis Conference in Arlington, Virginia, in 1990. Cited in "It's Important, but Don't Bank on Exercise Alone to Prevent Osteoporosis, Experts Say," Journal of the American Medical Association, April 4, 1990, p. 175.

[4] "Bone Savers: Rating Lifestyle and Drugs," Science News, October 21, 1991, p. 262.

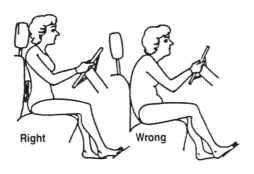

Right   Wrong

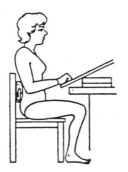

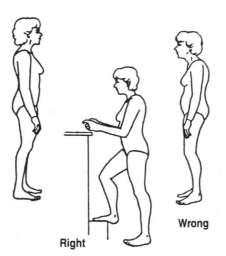

Right   Wrong

1. Sitting

When sitting, always use a rolled towel or bolster pillow two to four inches thick behind your lower back to aid in support. While driving, use the neck rest—increasing the thickness of the cushion slightly, if necessary—to support the natural curve of your neck.

When reading, do not lean over toward your work, but maintain the natural curvature of your back. At a desk, prop up a clipboard so it slants towards you, like a drafting table.

For relief after sitting for a while, do some postural exercises, such as the Wall Arch, Standing Back Bend, or Prone Press-Ups; these are illustrated in the next section, "Postural Exercises."

2. Standing

Keep your head high, chin in, shoulder blades slightly "pinched." Maintain the natural arch for your lower back.

While standing in one place for longer than a few minutes, put one foot up on a stool or in an open cupboard. Switch to the other foot periodically. You'll find this much less straining.

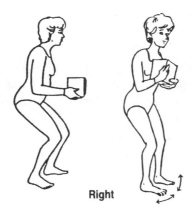

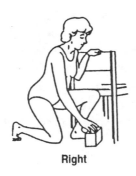

Right

Right

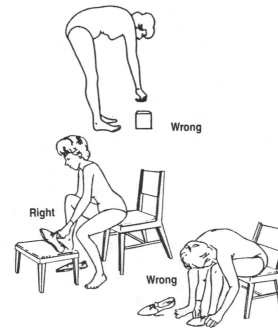

Wrong

Right

Wrong

3. Bending and Lifting

Keep your feet flat and in place; about shoulder width apart from one another. Both arms should touch your ribs or thighs, unless you're using one hand for support. As you bend, remember to maintain your natural low-back curve. Keep at least one foot flat on the ground to keep equal force at the hip, knee, and ankle. Gently breathe in while you are lifting the object or straightening up. When you reach an erect position, exhale.

When changing the direction you're facing, move your feet with your body. Pivot on your heels or toes with your knees slightly bent.

Never bend over to pick up an object forcing your back to be parallel to the ground. This position places a great deal of stress on your back.

These principles are important in all bending situations. As the bottom left illustration shows, whenever you need to bend over (for example, to tie your shoes, dry your feet, or shave your legs), maintain your natural low-back curve and flat upper back. Even when brushing your teeth, try not to bend from the waist, but rather bend at the knees.

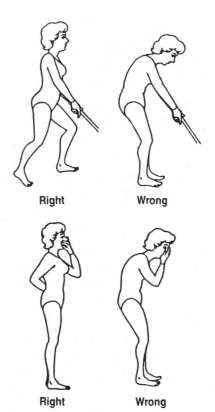

Right   Wrong

Right   Wrong

4. Pushing and Pulling

Instead of bending and twisting when you vacuum (or rake, sweep, etc.) use a foot-to-foot rocking movement. With knees bent and shoulder blades pinched, move forward and back, or side to side, rhythmically.

5. Coughing and Sneezing

Develop the habit of supporting your back with one hand whenever you cough or sneeze. This protects the spine and discs (tough cushions of cartilage between the nonfused vertebrae that act as shock absorbers) from damage caused by a sudden bend forward.

Postural Exercises

If you have a posture problem, you should get help from a physical therapist before starting the program shown here. The therapist will tailor the exercises to suit your needs. Individuals with decreased bone density or osteoporosis should avoid any unnecessary forward bending during daily activities —such as putting on shoes or vacuuming. Also, exercises that involve forward bending (eg, sit-ups or toe-touches) should be avoided because they can lead to crush fractures in the spine.

All of the following exercises have been designed for most individuals who already suffer from osteoporosis; however, in persons with extremely low bone density, these exercises should not be done. Always consult with your doctor before beginning an active exercise program.

We recommend that you begin with three repetitions. Work up to 10, by adding one a day. After a period of weeks, you will most likely find that you can readily do the entire program. The aim of these exercises is to direct you into a life of movement, in which physical activity is highly pleasurable to you. If any of these exercises cause pain or discomfort, omit them from your program.

1. Erect Walking

Walk with your chin in, head held high and shoulder blades slightly pinched. Wear shoes with rubber—or other nonslip—soles when walking and land lightly on your heels. Make sure your knee is lined up over your second toe at all times.

Practice with and without a towel roll on your head.

2. Wall Arch

Face a wall or doorway, stretching your arms up while taking a deep breath in. Concentrate on flattening your upper back. Also try reaching up with one arm while stretching down with the other.

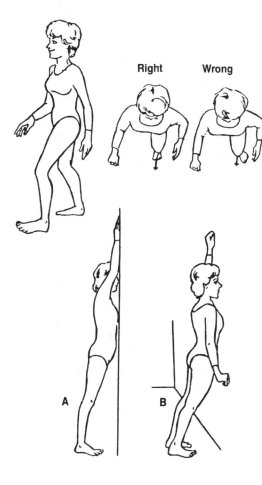

Right   Wrong

A   B

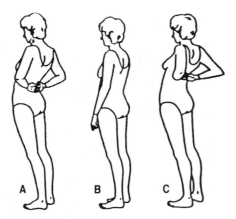

3. Standing Back Bend
Put your two fists on your lower back. Arch backwards slowly, while taking a deep breath. Repeat, placing the fists this time on the middle back. Repeat again with fists on the upper back.

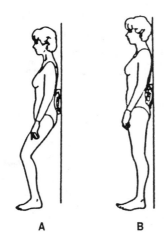

4. Wall Standing and Pelvic Tilt
Place your feet 12 inches away from a wall. With bent knees, have your head, shoulders, and upper back touching the wall. Use a towel roll at the level of your waist to support your lower back. This maneuver requires the use of the thigh, stomach, and spinal muscles.

Slide up and down, bending the knees and keeping the back flat. As you improve, you should be able to plant your feet closer to the wall while keeping your stomach muscles contracted.

5. Chin Pulls
Pull your chin in, as if you could move it to the back of your neck. Look straight forward, not up or down. Keep your head high. You will feel a stretch in the back of your neck and a flattening of your upper back. Push down on your knees to help your back become as erect as possible.

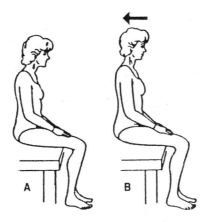

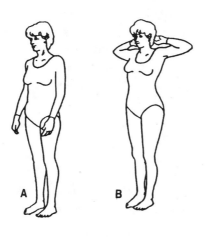

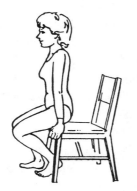

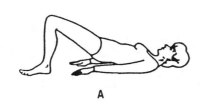

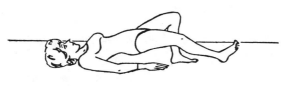

6. Isometric Posture Correction

Stand as tall as you can with your chin in, not up. Place your palms against the back of your head. Push against your scalp while simultaneously pinching your shoulder blades together. Build up a "resistance" to the count of three. After holding for three seconds, slowly release over three more seconds. Maintain an erect posture throughout this exercise.

7. Sitting Push-Ups

Sit near the edge of your chair using your hands for extra support. Lean forward. Lift the weight of your body as high as you comfortably can by straightening your arms and pushing up. Your feet should stay on the floor. Breathe in as you lift, exhale as you relax. Maintain the curvature of your lower back.

8. The Bridge

Lie on your back, keeping your knees bent. Press your head and shoulders down. Lift trunk, hips, and thighs. Relax. Repeat. As you improve, do with one leg only (alternating left and right leg).

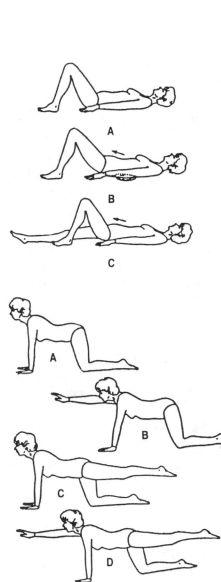

9. Pelvic Tilt With Leg Slide

Lie on your back with knees bent and a towel roll under your lower back. Press your back into the towel roll using your lower abdominal muscles and lifting your buttocks (not your whole back).

Slide one leg as far as you can, maintaining the tilt. Return to original position, relaxing the tilt. Repeat with the other leg.

10. All Fours Arm/Leg Lifts

Get on your hands and knees. Hands should be directly under the shoulders; knees should be directly under hips. Your back should be flat or slightly arched, as shown. Alternate lifting each arm, holding for three seconds. Then, alternate lifting each leg, holding for three seconds. If you can do this comfortably, lift your right arm and left leg simultaneously. Then alternate: lift left arm, right leg. Follow by sitting back on heels and stretching both arms forward as you exhale.

11. Prone Arm/Leg Lifts

Lift one arm from the shoulder and hold for three seconds. Relax. Repeat with the other arm. Then, lift one leg from the hip and hold for three seconds. Relax. Repeat with the other leg.

Lift the right arm and the left leg simultaneously and hold for three seconds. Relax. Repeat with the opposite arm and leg.

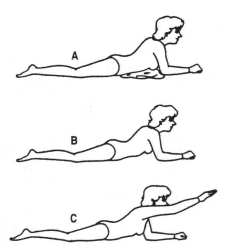

12. The Elbow Prop
As an alternative to sitting or lying on your back, try this position with or without a pillow. Attempt to stay in this position for one-half hour a day—starting at five minutes initially—while watching television or reading. By passively decompressing the vertebrae and discs, this position helps reverse damage caused by poor posture. A good back exercise in this position is to reach each arm forward, alternating left and right arms.

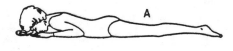

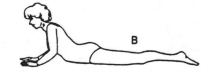

13. Prone Press-Ups With Deep Breathing
Start out in a conventional "push-up" position. Arch your back, pinching your shoulder blades together. As you raise up, inhale; as you go down, exhale. Keep elbows partially bent to protect the back. Use a pillow under your stomach for comfort, if necessary. Make sure you don't lift your pelvis.

SUMMING UP

Reviewing this step is easy: Get at least three to four hours a week of weight-bearing exercise, such as brisk walking, running, tennis, or aerobic dance.

CHAPTER FIVE

STEP FOUR—TAKE THE APPROPRIATE

DRUG THERAPY AS PRESCRIBED

BY A PHYSICIAN

Step four of osteoporosis prevention is to take the appropriate medications, prescribed by physicians, that prevent bone loss. This chapter covers the connection between estrogen and osteoporosis in women and other medications to prevent osteoporosis that are important to both women and men.

OSTEOPOROSIS AND ESTROGEN

You may have read or heard that osteoporosis is a woman's problem. This is not totally true. Men can and do develop weak bones. However, women are far more likely to have weak bones, primarily due to development of Type I osteoporosis, caused by loss of estrogen.

There is a direct link between low estrogen and bone loss. In industrialized countries women lose about 15 percent of their bone mass during the 15 years following menopause (when estrogen levels drop).[1] And 20 to 25 percent of postmenopausal women are at risk of suffering a fracture due to bone loss.[2]

A 1990 article in the prestigious Journal of the American Medical Association (JAMA) states that bone loss begins when low estrogen occurs and "irreplaceable bone has been lost by the time 3 years have passed."[3] The authors were referring to loss of estrogen due to overexercising. However, the loss also may result from a naturally occurring menopause or hysterectomy in which the ovaries are removed.

Here are accounts told to me by four women, all of whom say that taking estrogen has made a tremendous difference in their lives.

---

[1] "Osteoporosis," World Health, July-August 1991, p. 4.

[2] Ruth Papazian, "Osteoporosis Treatment Advances," FDA Consumer Magazine Reprint, April 1991.

[3] Mona Shangold et al., "Evaluation and Management of Menstrual Dysfunction in Athletes," Journal of the American Medical Association, March 23-30, 1990, p. 1667.

Sarah was born with only one kidney, and consequently as a child her doctor advised her not to drink milk. By age 47 she had two serious compression fractures in her spine, causing severe pain. First, she went to an orthopedic physician who told her that there wasn't anything he could do for her. Finally, she saw a specialist who put her on hormones for menopause and calcium supplements. Sarah has been on hormones for two years and has not had further fractures. A recent absorptiometry test showed improvement in her bone density.

. . .

Nora is 75 years old. Nine years ago she was helping her husband push his car and broke several vertebrae. Her doctor did not put her on hormones, but prescribed fluoride and calcium. The fractures and pain continued. Finally, after two years of constant pain, she started hormone therapy. She has not had a problem since.

. . .

Twenty years ago, at age 45, Betty had a hysterectomy. Her doctor did not recommend estrogen, saying "if you can get along without it, it would be better." She then had ten terrible years of back pain, as a number of her vertebrae compressed. Over the decade she lost 2 inches of height.

Finally, Betty went to a woman doctor who said, "Any doctor who said you shouldn't take estrogen should have to live with one who isn't taking it." Betty marvels that estrogen is the closest thing to the fountain of youth she has ever seen. She says, "I've gained tremendous relief from the constant pain I was in."

Estrogen has also had another major benefit for Betty. Prior to starting hormone therapy, she had such bad insomnia that she averaged only about three hours of sleep a night. Once on hormones, her sleeplessness went away.

During a telephone interview, Betty added the following: "Please put this in your report. I have a friend who is taking an entirely natural approach to menopause and refuses to take estrogen. I have watched her shrink and shrink."

• • •

Theresa is now 78. During her 70th year, she fractured a number of vertebrae over several months and became

slightly stooped. After the sixth vertebrae collapsed she went to the Mayo Clinic, where she
started using estrogen patches and had intense
physical therapy. The combination stopped progression of the disease.

As these four women's stories demonstrate, there is a
magic pill that can head off osteoporosis for women. If
you are near or through menopause, estrogen replacement
therapy (ERT) is by far the single most important measure
you can take to prevent Type I osteoporosis. In fact,
for most women, not taking estrogen is equivalent to
inviting your bones to disintegrate.

Anecdotal information and numerous scientific studies
have shown that estrogen prevents osteoporosis in
midlife and older women. Researchers think that
estrogen works by returning bone resorption and
formation rates to the right balance. It is known that
estrogen works directly on bone cells that have
estrogen "receptors."

An expert panel convened by the National Institutes of
Health and the American Medical Association (AMA)
pinpointed estrogen as the best deterrent to osteoporo-

sis in women. Here is what the AMA has to say about estrogen and osteoporosis:

"Treatment is most effective when given before significant bone loss has occurred and has been shown to delay bone loss for at least eight years.

. . . When estrogen treatment is withdrawn, bone loss resumes.[4]

Here is more proof of the benefits of estrogen:

- An article in the New England Journal of Medicine states that, for women with osteoporosis, estrogen therapy increases bone mass by 5 percent and cuts the risk of vertebrae fractures in half.[5]

- A ten-year study at Goldwater Memorial Hospital in New York found that women who take estrogen

---

[4] Council on Scientific Affairs, "Estrogen Replacement in the Menopause," Journal of the American Medical Association, January 21, 1983, p. 359.

[5] B. Lawrence Riggs and L. Joseph Melton, "The Prevention and Treatment of Osteoporosis," New England Journal of Medicine, August 27, 1992, p. 620.

after menopause do not develop osteoporosis, while those who do not take it do.

- Another study found that estrogen replacement therapy cuts the risk of hip fractures in half. In yet another long term study, 1,000 women treated for 15 years with estrogen reduced wrist fractures by 70 percent. And no hip fractures occurred among these women in the 15 years.

Sadly, although 95 percent of older women would benefit from estrogen replacement therapy, only 15 percent are receiving it.[6] The protective effects of estrogen are particularly important to the 50 million women who will go through menopause in the next ten years.

There is evidence that estrogen in combination with progesterone, now the standard form of treatment for

---

[6] Andrew Skolnick, "At Third Meeting, Menopause Experts Make the Most of Insufficient Data," Journal of the American Medical Association, November 11, 1992, p. 2508.

menopausal symptoms, may promote formation of new bone.[7] In one study conducted by Dr. Lila Nachtigall, a well-known expert on menopause, for women who took estrogen and progesterone less than three years after the onset of their menopause, bone density increased over the course of the ten-year period. This was not the case for women who were not on the combination therapy.[8] Other studies have confirmed this finding.

Hormones are also important to young women who are still developing peak bone mass. Bone mass increases with the use of oral contraceptives.[9]

---

[7] R. Don Gambrell, "Update on Hormone Replacement Therapy," American Family Physician, November 1992, p. 88S.

[8] L. E. Nachtigall et al., "Estrogen Replacement Therapy: A 10 Year Prospective Study in the Relationship to Osteoporosis," Obstetrics and Gynecology, Vol. 53, 1979, pp. 277-281.

[9] R. R. Recker, "Bone Gain in Young Adult Women," Journal of the American Medical Association, November 4, 1992, p. 2403.

<u>How to Tell if You Are in Menopause</u>

It is important to detect when you are in the early stages of menopause because most bone is lost in the first three to six years after it begins.[10] Most women eventually experience at least three or four of the major signs of menopause listed next. If this is the case for you, be sure to see your doctor who will give you a blood test to determine if you should take estrogen:[11]

Hot flashes or flushes

Changes in menstruation

Vaginal changes

Stress incontinence

Weight gain

---

[10] B. Lawrence Riggs and L. Joseph Melton, "The Prevention and Treatment of Osteoporosis," <u>New England Journal of Medicine</u>, August 27, 1992, p. 620.

[11] The blood test to determine if estrogen replacement is necessary is called a FSH (for follicle stimulating hormone) level. If the FSH level is high estrogen should be started. (FSH levels increase when estrogen levels dip.)

Skin and hair changes

Premenstrual syndrome

Sleep changes

Mood swings

Although less common, other symptoms can occur before and during menopause. They include migraine headaches, dizziness, heart palpitations, aching joints, cold hands and feet (regardless of the weather), fatigue, lethargy, jitters, shortness of breath, and a feeling that there are insects crawling all over the body.

What Is the Best Dosage for Estrogen?

Estrogen in minimum doses of 0.625 mg a day will prevent osteoporosis from developing in 90 percent of women who have passed menopause.[12] Hormone therapy should be started immediately when estrogen levels begin to decline. However, it is still effective if begun later. Estrogen therapy must be continued to prevent bone loss. If you stop taking it, your bone mass will begin to decrease.

---

[12] Gambrell, "Update on Hormone Replacement Therapy," p. 89S.

If you already have osteoporosis, you may need to take a higher dosage of estrogen than that mentioned to prevent further development of the condition.

It Is Never Too Late to Start Estrogen

A study conducted at the Mayo Clinic found estrogen to be effective for prevention and treatment of osteoporosis even up to 75 years of age. In fact, it cuts in half the chance of fracture in patients who have already developed osteoporosis.[13]

If Your Ovaries Have Been Removed

If you have had a total hysterectomy, you should be taking estrogen, unless another health condition prevents it. This is true regardless of your age or whether you have any symptoms.

When Not to Take Estrogen

In the past, many women were afraid to take hormones, and many physicians were reluctant to prescribe them.

---

[13] "Estrogen and Osteoporosis, Reevaluating the Timetable, Emergency Medicine, October 15, 1992, p. 275.

The result was that many women developed osteoporosis, along with other conditions such as heart disease. Now, in the 1990s, the standard of treatment has changed dramatically, because, for most women, the consequences of <u>not</u> taking estrogen are <u>far greater</u> than the risks of taking it.

On the other hand, if you have any of the following health conditions, estrogen replacement therapy is not for you:

- A history of estrogen-dependent tumors of the breast or lining of the uterus

- Problems with blood clots (thrombophlebitis or thromboembolism)

- Severe liver disease[14]

In addition, if you smoke, or have any of the following your physician should carefully monitor your estrogen replacement therapy:

---

[14] Robert Berkow, ed., <u>The Merck Manual of Diagnosis and Therapy</u>, 15th ed., (New Jersey: Merck, Sharpe and Doehme Research Laboratories, 1987), pp. 1714-1715.

- fibroid tumors

- bleeding between periods

- obesity

- diabetes

- hypertension

- gallbladder disease

You also should not take estrogen if you are pregnant or are breast feeding. Estrogen therapy during pregnancy increases the risk of birth defects. Breast-feeding mothers should not take estrogen because it passes into breast milk.

Other Advantages of Taking Estrogen

If you can take estrogen you will not only have stronger bones, but most menopausal symptoms also will be eliminated or greatly reduced. Symptoms include:

- Hot flashes

- Sleeplessness or insomnia

- Lack of desire for sex

- Deterioration of organs and tissues such as genital and urinary organs

In addition, estrogen has other dramatic benefits for your health, quality of life, and longevity. Most notably, your chances of developing any of the following health problems will be dramatically lessened: heart disease, stroke, and urinary incontinence (which is surprisingly common). However, many women have fears about taking estrogen.

Here is a summary of the pros and cons of taking estrogen, from my book <u>Keys to Menopause and Beyond</u>.[15]

<u>Pros</u>

> <u>General health:</u> Women who do <u>not</u> take estrogen are <u>three</u> times more likely to die of all causes.
>
> <u>Coronary heart disease:</u> Reduces risk 44 to 51 percent.
>
> <u>Strokes:</u> Reduces risk 30 percent or more.
>
> <u>Bone thinning (osteoporosis):</u> Significant reduction in risk.
>
> <u>Vagina and vulva:</u> Restored to normal.

———————————————————

[15] Elizabeth Vierck, <u>Keys to Menopause and Beyond</u>, (New York: Barron's, 1992), pp. 59-60.

Mood swings: Greatly reduced.

Hot Flashes: Greatly reduced.

Sexual intercourse: Restores comfort and, therefore, pleasure; restores libido.

Skin: Moisture restored and firmer.

Muscles: Firmer and stronger.

Hair: Stronger.

Breasts: Firmer.

Arthritis: Some studies have shown that estrogen relieves arthritic pain and reduces the incidence of rheumatoid arthritis.

Snoring: Eliminated.

Sleep problems: Greatly reduced.

Cons

Hypertension: One in 20 women has a rise in blood pressure. By using estrogen vaginal cream or the transdermal skin patch in place of a tablet, the problem can be side-stepped.

Gallstones: Affects bile in the liver. By using estrogen vaginal cream or the transdermal skin patch in place of a tablet, the problem can be side-stepped.

Fibroids: Fibroid tumors can proliferate.

Expense: Hormone replacement therapy has a high annual cost and must be taken for life to maintain benefits.

Concerns

Breast cancer: Although it does not appear to cause breast cancer, estrogen may promote the growth of preexisting tumors. Some studies have shown it to be protective against breast cancer. Others have found it to be a risk for women who take it for a long time.

Uterine cancer: No increased risk when used with progesterone. It may, however, make already existing cancers grow faster.

Note: Supporting data for these pros and cons are found in the following sources: Lila E. Nachtigall and Joan Rattner Heilman, Estrogen, (New York: Harper Perennial, 1991); Council on Scientific Affairs, "Estrogen Replacement in the Menopause," <u>Journal of the American Medical Association</u>, January 21, 1983; American Cancer Society, <u>Cancer Facts and Figures</u> (Georgia ACS, 1992); Robert Berkow, ed., <u>The Merck Manual of Diagnosis and Therapy</u>, 15th ed. (New Jersey: Merck, Sharpe and Doehme Research Laboratories, 1987); Morton A. Stenchever and George Aagaard, <u>Caring for the Older Woman</u> (New York: Elsevier, 1991); and Dr. Lawrence Scrima, Rose Sleep Disorders Center, Denver, Colorado.

<u>How to Take Estrogen</u>

Estrogen is taken most often in pill form, and Premarin™ is prescribed most frequently. The minimal effective dosage is 0.625 mg. Except for women who have had their uterus removed, progesterone is usually taken along with estrogen to reduce or eliminate the risk of cancer of the uterus.

Research conducted by Dr. Jerilynn Prior at the University of British Columbia in Vancouver suggests that taking progesterone provides additional protection against osteoporosis. Dr. Prior found that women with low levels of progesterone lost bone. She also says that there is a lot of evidence that progesterone spurs the growth of new bone.[16]

While side effects are not common, you may experience any of the following symptoms for a couple of months after starting estrogen therapy: salt and water retention causing bloating, weight gain, breast swelling and tenderness, headaches, nausea, vomiting, dizziness, and vaginal infections. These side effects should go away, or you and your doctor should discuss changing your dosage.

As of this writing, there are four major ways that you can take estrogen and progesterone. You should discuss these with your doctor to decide which one is the best for you:

- Mimicking the menstrual cycle—estrogen every day of the month and progestin for 12 to 14 days.

- Five to nine days off hormones—estrogen for 21 to 25 days in combination with progestin for 7 to 12 of those days.

---

[16] "Menstrual Glitches May Spur Bone Loss," Science News, November 3, 1990, p. 279.

- <u>Continuous ERT</u>—estrogen and a low dose of progestin daily.

- <u>Taking estrogen alone</u>—this method is for women who have had their uteruses removed; estrogen alone is taken daily.

Estrogen Patches

Estrogen is available in a patch. However, a warning is in order. The patch may not protect against osteoporosis as reliably as the estrogen pill. You may want to stick with estrogen pills until more information is available on the effectiveness of the estrogen patch where osteoporosis is concerned.

Estrogen Is Not the Bottom Line

While estrogen is vitally important for women who want to prevent osteoporosis, it is not the bottom line. Osteoporosis prevention is a four-step process—one step of which is taking hormone supplements when estrogen levels drop. Estrogen does a great job of protecting against one particular type of osteoporosis (Type I). However, women frequently develop other types of the disease, for example, Type II osteoporosis, which both men and women get.

If you are taking estrogen, that is great. You are doing yourself a huge favor. But don't be complacent. It is also important to be aware of any other risk factors you have, to perform weight-bearing exercise on a regular basis, and to follow the nutrition guidelines presented in Chapter Three of this report.

FOR WOMEN AND MEN: BONE-BUILDING MEDICATIONS

Janet, now age 52, went through menopause at age 42. She did not take hormones because of a strong family history of cancer. At about age 46 she had a bone density test as part of the requirement to enter a study on osteoporosis. Researchers found that she had the bones of an 80-year-old woman. Her bones were three deviations below normal.

Janet finally went to a specialist who put her on a medication called calcitonin. She also takes calcium, eats yogurt and drinks milk every day, and exercises religiously. She swims half a mile three days a week and works with weights two days a week to strengthen her supporting muscles. Last year her bones were tested and showed a significant 7 percent increase in density.

Janet is now without pain for the first time in 35 years. She reports with pride that she visited a friend recently whom she had not seen in a long time. Her friend said, "You look so different." "Why?" asked Janet. "Because of the lack of pain in your face," remarked the friend. She has had many other friends tell her that she looks much younger now that the pain is gone.

•   •   •

Sandra Wagner is now 67 and has had osteoporosis for about seven years. Sandra's diagnosis was a fluke. On a lark she accompanied a friend to a local health fair that was offering low-cost bone density analyses. Her friend turned out to be fine, but Sandra's bones were found to be "close to powder." Only luck had kept her from a serious fracture. Up to that point she had not noticed any symptoms. Sandra immediately went to a noted Denver specialist and, to her dismay, found that she had shrunk 1¼ inches.

Sandra tried every type of estrogen but could not tolerate it because of what it did to her breasts. She went from a padded bra to filling out a 38C, and her breasts were so painful that she could not take a shower without crying from the pain of the weight of the water. The specialist put her on an alternative medicine and calcium. She exercises three to five times a week and walks a great deal, doing 45 minutes on the treadmill on days when the weather is bad. Sandra has been able to halt progression of her osteoporosis even though she can't take estrogen.

As these two cases demonstrate, there are other important drugs, besides estrogen, that increase bone mass and prevent the pain, disability, and deformity of osteoporosis. If you are a man and are at high risk for osteoporosis or are a woman near or past menopause, but you cannot take estrogen, you should discuss taking one of these medications with your physician.

Several new drugs show great promise against osteoporosis. A drug called alendronate leads the pack because it is effective for several different types of bone, including hip bone. Up to this point no other drug, outside of estrogen, had been shown to be effective against the wasting of hip bone.

At this time, the government has approved only estrogen and calcitonin to prevent osteoporosis. However, your doctor can prescribe other medications for osteoporosis prevention as he or she sees fit. Here is a breakdown of the most important medications available for osteoporosis prevention.

PROVEN BONE BUILDERS

Calcitonin

If you are postmenopausal and cannot take estrogen, you should probably be using calcitonin to ward off osteoporosis. Calcitonin is a hormone that occurs naturally in the body and affects internal calcium regulation.

Calcitonin is the best option available for women who cannot take estrogen. It works by decreasing bone demolition. It is particularly effective for Type I osteoporosis and has added benefits of reducing pain and increasing mobility. For women who can take estrogen, some osteoporosis experts feel that estrogen given together with calcitonin may be particularly effective.

Calcitonin is now available only through injection. (Tablets are not effective, because the hormone is not compatible with gastrointestinal juices.) Unhappily, it is expensive. A nasal spray is being developed, which may be easier to use and more affordable. The hormone can cause mild side effects, including flushing, nausea, vomiting, diarrhea, and abdominal cramps. However, side effects are rarely severe enough to stop use of the drug.

Unfortunately, there are some drawbacks to calcitonin, and there is some debate about how long it is effective. Studies are now taking place to investigate the long-term effectiveness of the drug. For unknown reasons, some people do not respond to the drug.

Bisphosphonates

Bisphosphonates are presently receiving a great deal of attention for their potential in preventing and treating osteoporosis. They work by reducing bone loss (resorption) and the occurrence of vertebrae fractures. Perhaps the best known bisphosphonate is etridonate. The drug is particularly beneficial for prevention of spinal fractures. It actually increases bone density of the spine. However, it may not be effective against other types of fractures.[17] Patients take etridonate for 2 weeks every 2 to 3 months and calcium for 11 weeks of

---

[17] Gambrell, "Update on Hormone Replacement Therapy," p. 88S.

each cycle. Only 5 percent to 6 percent of patients have side effects, which are usually minimal.

Patients at the Osteoporosis Prevention Center in Decatur, Georgia, have taken etridonate since 1985 with impressive results. Severely debilitated patients have returned to normal, and patients continually gain bone density in the spine.[18] Etridonate also relieves pain from small fractures. Other studies have had similar results.

Etridonate appears to continue to increase bone mass after two years of therapy. And there are no known disadvantages to taking it. Etridonate will not put a strain on your pocketbook. On average, it costs about $12 a month.

Researchers are testing bisphosphonates further. A recent article in Geriatrics magazine reports that the

---

[18] Grattan C. Woodson et al., "Treating Osteoporosis," Senior Patient, March-April 1991, p. 8.

bisphosphonate <u>alendronate</u> increased lumbar spine, hip bone, and total skeletal bone density during recent research trials.[19] This is an important breakthrough. Other research has pinpointed drugs that increase density of the lumbar spine, but not hip bone and total skeletal density. Six thousand patients now are taking alendronate in a four-year study to further evaluate its effects.

Parathyroid Hormone

Parathyroid hormone increases bone formation when given in low dosages. It is currently being studied for effectiveness against osteoporosis.

Thiazides

Researchers are now looking into the benefit of a class of diuretics that promote excretion by the kidneys called thiazides. Thiazides reduce the loss of calcium in

---

[19] "Drug Research: Agents Show Promise for Osteoporosis, CNS Injury," <u>Geriatrics</u>, Vol. 48, No. 1, January 1993, p. 21.

urination. A recent study found that taking thiazides can reduce risk of hip fracture by one-third.[20] Other types of diuretics have not been found to be effective against bone loss.

Testosterone for Men

Decreases in male hormones can cause bone loss and osteoporosis. The National Osteoporosis Foundation asserts that, when fractures occur in older men, decreasing hormones are usually the cause. The number of men with osteoporosis is growing. In fact, men are the victims of almost a third of all hip fractures and another 13 percent of all spinal fractures.[21] If you are a male and you have symptoms of osteoporosis, you may want to discuss testosterone treatments with your physician.[22]

---

[20] Andrea LaCroix et al., "Thiazide Diuretic Agents and the Incidence of Hip Fracture," New England Journal of Medicine, February 1, 1990, p. 286.

[21] "Osteoporosis: Not for Women Only," Arthritis Today, March 1993, p. 13.

[22] R. M. Francis et al., "Osteoporosis in Hypogonadal Men," Bone, Vol. 7, 1986, pp. 261-268.

OTHER MEDICATIONS AND TECHNIQUES

Other medications and techniques such as fluoride, steroids, and electrical stimulation are frequently mentioned as remedies for osteoporosis. However, they have not been found to be as desirable as the medications mentioned earlier, or they are experimental at this point and are not available to the health consumer. Here are brief descriptions of the major drugs and techniques you may have heard about.

Sodium Fluoride

Dentists have used sodium fluoride for years to strengthen teeth. At one time it was the great hope for osteoporosis victims because it clearly increases bone mass. However, fluoride therapy causes irregular and inferior bone growth. The result is that the skeleton becomes <u>more</u> fragile. Side effects include pain in the large joints, nausea, vomiting, and hemorrhage.

Anabolic Steroids (Androgens)

Anabolic steroids are the drugs that weight lifters use to build up their muscles. While they may be useful

112

in preventing bone loss, masculinizing side effects make these drugs an unrealistic choice for women.

Calcitriol

Calcitriol, the active component of vitamin D, has been found to be more effective than calcium supplements in preventing fractures in women who have osteoporosis. There is no difference in terms of side effects.[23] Calcitriol works by promoting calcium absorption and stimulating bone-building cells. Too much calcitriol can cause an overdose of vitamin D. Unfortunately, at this time calcitriol is not available in the United States for the treatment of osteoporosis.

Tamoxifen

Tamoxifen has been used since 1971 in women with breast cancer to prevent cancer in the other breast. An added benefit of tamoxifen is that it may also reduce the risk of heart disease and osteoporosis. However, the side effects do not make it practical to use for osteoporosis prevention alone, because there are other options available.

---

[23] Research conducted by Murray W. Tilyard and coworkers, University of Otago, Dunedin, New Zealand.

Human Growth Hormone

Human growth hormone is now used to treat children who are not growing normally. Researchers are studying its benefits for healing hip fractures and preventing and treating osteoporosis. The hormone is expensive and has serious side effects, which make it impractical at this time.

Jolting Bone Density

Researchers are presently studying painless doses of electricity to prevent or treat osteoporosis. In animal studies physiologists Clinton Rubin and Kenneth McLeod at the State University of New York at Stony Brook found that small doses of electricity increased bone mass by 12 percent in two months. Rubin is now conducting a two-year study on 20 postmenopausal women to see if the electrical current is as successful with humans. If so, portable electrical outlets may be available soon to ward off bone loss.

MEDICATIONS THAT TREAT MEDICAL CONDITIONS
THAT LEAD TO OSTEOPOROSIS

It is important to take the prescribed medications to treat any health condition such as diabetes that can lead to osteoporosis. For information about the medical conditions that cause osteoporosis, see Chapter Three.

SUMMING UP

If you are a woman in your forties, begin hormone replacement therapy when estrogen levels begin to decline, unless you have a medical condition that prevents it. If you are older and are not on estrogen, seriously consider taking it.

If you are a woman near or past menopause, but you cannot take estrogen, or you are a man who is at high risk for osteoporosis, you should consider taking one of the drugs that increases bone mass and prevents the pain, disability, and deformity of osteoporosis. In addition, if you have one of the medical conditions that leads to osteoporosis, it is important to take the prescribed medications for your condition to prevent bone loss.

A REVIEW OF THE FOUR STEPS
TO OSTEOPOROSIS PREVENTION

By following these steps, you can prevent osteoporosis or slow down its progression if it has already started. You may want to make a copy of this page and keep it with your personal papers as a reminder.

1. <u>Learn about the risk factors for osteoporosis</u>. The more risk factors you have, the greater your chances for developing weak bones.

2. <u>Develop a well-rounded, high-calcium diet</u>. Think calcium, get adequate vitamin D, and cut down on foods that block calcium absorption.

3. <u>Get plenty of weight-bearing exercise</u>. Get at least three to four hours of weight-bearing exercise a week. Walk, run, play tennis, dance, exercise!

4. <u>Take the appropriate drug therapy as prescribed by a physician</u>. If you are a woman in your forties, begin hormone replacement therapy when estrogen levels begin to decline. If you cannot take estrogen or are a high-risk male, take bone-building medications such as calcitonin as prescribed by a physician. Take the appropriate medications to treat medical conditions such as diabetes that can lead to osteoporosis.

CHAPTER SIX

LIVING WITH OSTEOPOROSIS—HOW TO PREVENT INJURY

Even minor mishaps can result in a serious fracture if you have osteoporosis. Consider these facts:

- Falls are the leading cause of accidental death among older people and are a significant cause among younger people.

- Most falls occur in the home.

- Falls are the major cause of admission of one-third of residents in nursing homes.

Often just being aware of danger helps you avoid it. Take this advice from the National Institutes of Health (NIH):

Prevention of falls is especially important for people who have osteoporosis. Falls and accidents seldom "just happen," and many can be prevented.

The following are some guidelines from NIH for preventing falls and fractures:

- Have your vision and hearing tested regularly and properly corrected. Have cataract surgery performed if necessary. Even the simple act of removing ear wax can improve your balance.

- Talk to your doctor or pharmacist about the side effects of the drugs you are taking and how they may affect your coordination or balance. Ask them to suggest ways to reduce the possibilities for falling.

- Limit your intake of alcohol. Even a little alcohol can further disturb already impaired balance and reflexes.

- Use caution in getting up too quickly after eating, lying down, or resting. Low blood pressure may cause dizziness at these times.

- Make sure that the nighttime temperature in your home is not lower than 65° Fahrenheit. Prolonged exposure to cold temperatures may cause body temperatures to drop, leading to dizziness and falling.

- Use a cane, walking stick, or walker to help maintain balance on uneven or unfamiliar ground or if you sometimes feel dizzy. Use special caution in walking outdoors on wet and icy pavement.

- Wear supportive, rubber-soled, low-heeled shoes. Avoid wearing only socks or smooth-soled shoes or slippers on stairs or waxed floors. They make it very easy to slip.

- Maintain a regular program of exercise. Regular physical activity improves strength and muscle tone, which will help in moving about more easily by keeping joints, tendons, and ligaments more flexible. It is important, however, to check with your doctor or physical therapist to plan a suitable exercise program.

In addition, follow these tips to avoid spinal fractures:

- Learn how to lift without straining the back.

- Avoid forceful movements.

- Use handles with long arms to lift things in and out of the oven or reach things in shelves, lubricate windows so they don't get stuck, and use assistive devices such as those mentioned in the section beginning on page 125.

SAFETY BEGINS AT HOME

The following is a safety checklist for your home, compliments of the National Institutes of Health.

Check to see that

Stairways, hallways, and pathways have

- Good lighting and are free of clutter.

- Firmly attached carpet, rough texture, or abrasive strips to secure footing.

- Tightly fastened handrails running the entire length and along both sides of all stairs, with light switches at the top and bottom.

Bathrooms have

- Grab bars conveniently located in and out of tubs and showers and near toilets.

- Nonskid mats, abrasive strips, or carpet on all surfaces that may get wet.

- Nightlights.

Bedrooms have

- Nightlights or light switches within reach of bed(s).

- Easily reached telephones, convenient to the bed(s).

Living areas have

- Electrical cords and telephone wires placed out of walking paths.

- Rugs well secured to the floor.

- Furniture (especially low coffee tables) and other objects arranged so they are not in the way.

- Couches and chairs at proper height to get into and out of easily.

In addition,

Throughout the house

- All rugs are secure and will not slip and slide. Do not use throw rugs!

- Make sure that all cords or anything similar you could trip over are out of the way, wherever you walk. Watch out for children's and pets' toys.

- Make sure that all areas that you walk through are well lighted, including those outside the house.

NEW RESEARCH ON PREVENTING FALLS

Several research centers are studying how to prevent and decrease the damage from falls. They include the National Institutes of Health in Washington, D.C., the National Research Council in Chicago, Illinois, and the Safe Program (Study to Assess Falls Among the Elderly) at The Centers for Disease Control in Atlanta, Georgia. Many of these studies are looking at ways to improve stairs and railings to prevent falls.

Another approach is preventing injury when an individuals falls, rather than preventing the fall itself. Dr. David Colvin, president of the Triangle Research and Development Corporation in Research Triangle Park, North Carolina, has devised a number of products to reduce injury. One, called Fall-Safe, is presently being tested in a nursing home in Maryland. It is most beneficial for elderly individuals who are limited and confined. Patients wear a vest, which is attached to an overhead track. If they fall, the system catches them and absorbs most of the shock, while gently lowering them to the floor. A major benefit of the system is older men and women get more exercise, because wearing the system eliminates the fear of falling while walking.

Another project Colvin is working on is air bags to protect hips and knees. They are similar to life jackets. Inserted in garments, they have sensors that detect when the wearer is about to fall, and they release a cushioning gas into the garment around the knees and hips.

ASSISTIVE DEVICES

Assistive devices work by helping osteoporosis victims prevent further injury and reduce pain. For example, if you have had significant spinal fractures and are experiencing low-back pain, you may have a condition called iliocostal friction syndrome (ICFS), which means that your ribs are touching a sensitive area of your body called the iliac crest. An important device that can provide relief from pain and prevent the need for surgery for the ICFS sufferer is an elastic belt that

compresses the lower ribs and removes them from contact
with the sensitive area.

Assistive devices are available from medical supply
stores and catalogs. Some products, such as the elastic
belt just described, can be made to your specifications
by local medical suppliers. Some devices are covered by
Medicare and other insurance plans. But check with your
insurance carrier first to make sure that the specific
item you are purchasing is reimbursable under its
guidelines.

Here is a highly selective list of assistive devices.
For a more complete and updated list contact Abledata,
listed in the appendix.

- Back supports and abdominal binders relieve pain
  of spinal fractures.

- Assisto-seats push you up and out of your chair.
  Portable models are available for increased
  mobility.

- Carts on wheels help move things from room to
  room.

- Pill box alarms keep track of medication times.

- <u>Reachers</u> grab items more than an arm's length away.

- <u>Dressing sticks</u> help pull on clothes.

- <u>Shoe removers</u> and <u>stocking helpers</u> assist with putting on and taking off shoes, stockings, and socks.

- <u>Velcro</u> can be artfully hidden behind buttons to make dressing easier.

- <u>Grab bars</u> provide safety when getting in and out of the bathtub or shower; they should be in every bathroom, regardless of the occupants' age.

- <u>Transfer benches</u> and <u>tub and shower benches</u> provide help for getting in and out of the tub and bathing.

- <u>Multipurpose commode chairs</u> with wheels are versatile for the homebound.

- <u>Glideabouts</u> or <u>three-wheeled motorized scooters</u> provide mobility for anyone with limited movement.

- <u>Walkers</u> come in a number of models, including folding, seated with wheels, and three wheeled.

CHAPTER SEVEN

OVERCOMING PAIN

Pain is the body's message that something is wrong. The pain of osteoporosis is usually the result of fractures and frequently is the first sign of the disease. The pain of osteoporosis can be acute, chronic, or both. It is subjective. Only the victim can describe it, and it varies by individual. The pain that may be unbearable to you may be but a twinge to another.

Acute pain is the most common and is usually treatable with medications, rest, and limiting activity. It is the type of pain that an osteoporosis sufferer experiences when breaking a hip or wrist. It is intense, but blessedly temporary. By definition, chronic pain is long term, lasting over six months. It is often a lifetime companion. Chronic pain often accompanies compression fractures of the spine and is harder to treat than acute pain. The following pages describe a number of measures to control both types of pain.

PAIN MEDICATIONS

Pain-killing drugs are called analgesics. They are narcotic or nonnarcotic. Narcotic pain killers block pain signals within the nervous system. They are habit forming and produce tolerance, which means that the user has to use increasing amounts over time to receive the same benefit. Nonnarcotic analgesics are less powerful but are not habit forming and do not cause tolerance. Most, with the exception of acetaminophen (Tylenol™), work by blocking nerve endings at the site of the pain.

The following describes the most common pain killers:

Aspirin is the most frequently taken drug in the world. It is a nonnarcotic drug that reduces pain and also helps cut down on inflammation. Aspirin is affordable for most health consumers. However, it can be very hard on the stomach. Frequent side effects include nausea, vomiting, abdominal pain, heartburn, and indigestion. Intestinal bleeding, ulcers, and allergic reactions also may occur.

Acetaminophen is often a better alternative than taking aspirin or related drugs that are hard on the stomach. In contrast to other pain killers, it is relatively free of side effects. It works by blocking pain signals at the nervous system level. However, too much acetamino- phen can damage the liver and kidneys. It reduces fever as well as pain. Common brand names for acetaminophen are Anacin-3™, Excedrin™, Tylenol™, and Vanquish™. Like

130

aspirin, acetaminophen is relatively inexpensive, particularly in generic form. Acetaminophen is <u>not</u> addic-
tive.

<u>Darvon™ (propoxyphene)</u> is used for the short-term
relief of pain. Because it is a narcotic, it is <u>not</u>
appropriate as part of a long-term treatment plan. It
may cause stomach upset.

<u>Codeine</u> is a narcotic pain reliever that provides help
against moderate pain. It is <u>not</u> appropriate as part of
a long-term treatment plan. Side effects include nausea,
constipation, dizziness, flushed face, difficulty in
urination, fatigue, and drowsiness.

<u>Nonsteroidal anti-inflammatory drugs (NSAIDs)</u> are mild
pain killers that also work against inflammation. There
are over 100 variations of NSAIDs internationally.
Gastrointestinal problems and allergic reactions can
occur. Most NSAIDs are available by prescription only.
Common NSAIDs include aspirin, ibuprofen, and naprosyn.

Analgesic ointments include Ben-Gay™, Aspercreme™, and
Tiger Balm™. They provide temporary, soothing relief to
sore spots by improving circulation to that area of the
body.

RULES OF DRUG USE

Taking pain medication daily for osteoporosis has some risks, including allergic reactions, side effects, and accidental overdosing. The following basic rules of drug use from the National Institutes of Health reduce the risks that go along with taking these medications:

- Take exactly the amount of the drug prescribed by your doctor and follow the dosage schedule as closely as possible. If you have trouble or questions, call your doctor or pharmacist.

- Medicines do not produce the same effects in all people. Never take drugs prescribed for a friend or relative, even though your symptoms may be the same.

- Always tell your doctor about past problems you have had with drugs (such as rashes, indigestion, dizziness, or lack of appetite). When your doctor prescribes a new drug, be sure to mention all other medicines you are currently taking—including those prescribed by another doctor and those you buy without a prescription.

- Keep a daily record of the drugs you are taking, especially if your treatment schedule is complicated or you are taking more than one drug at a time. The record should show the name of the drug, the doctor who prescribed it, the amount you take, and the times of day for taking it. Keep a copy in your medicine cabinet and one in your wallet or pocketbook.

- If childproof containers are hard for you to handle, ask your pharmacist for easy-to-open containers. Always be sure, however, that they are out of the reach of children.

- Make sure that you understand the directions printed on the drug container and that the name of the medicine is clearly printed on the label. Ask your pharmacist to use large type on the label if you find the regular labels hard to read.

- Discard old medicines; many drugs lose their effectiveness over time.

- When you start taking a new drug, ask your doctor or pharmacist about side effects that may occur, about special rules for storage, and about foods or beverages, if any, to avoid. Pharmacists are able to answer most questions about drug use.

- Always call your doctor promptly if you notice unusual reactions.

- You should occasionally review with your doctor the need for each medicine that you are taking.

HOT AND COLD TREATMENTS

Hot and cold treatments can provide welcome relief for pain. Heat has been used for centuries for relieving pain. Application of heat (thermotherapy) increases the flow of blood to the affected area, soothing pain. Heat applications you might want to try include:

- Heat lamps, which provide penetrating heat to the affected area.

- Heating pads, available in both dry and dry/moist heat.

- Hot tubs and whirlpools.

- Hot water bottles.

- Warm towels.

Cold can reduce muscle spasms and stimulates the production of pain-relieving endorphins. Options include gel-type packs, plastic baggies with ice in them, or bags of frozen vegetables. Never place ice directly onto the skin.

R AND R—REST AND RELAXATION

Rest and relaxation can greatly reduce the perception of pain. For example, pain from compression fractures often creates tight muscles and anxiety. R and R can help relieve both. Here is a checklist of some popular rest and relaxation techniques.

Deep breathing is the oldest stress-reducing technique known to us. The phrase "Take a deep breath to calm down" originates with this technique. It involves breathing deeply and slowly from the diaphragm.

Autogenic relaxing involves talking yourself into relaxing. For example, you get comfortable and tell different parts of your body to relax: "My toes are now relaxed. The balls of my feet are now relaxed." The idea is to shut off conscious thoughts and free unconscious, healing thoughts.

135

Biofeedback uses equipment that monitors your physical reactions and gives you information on them. This technique is very useful for people who have a hard time knowing when their body is relaxed.

Imagery/creative visualization uses mental imagery to improve health and attitudes and block pain perception. You visualize a favorite place that is associated with peaceful feelings or make one up, such as floating on a cloud.

Meditation involves concentrating on one sound or thought to reach a relaxed, peaceful state.

Prayer, for many, is a way of relaxing and reaching a peaceful state of mind.

Progressive muscle relaxation teaches the difference between tight and relaxed muscles by alternately tensing and relaxing muscles.

Self-hypnosis is a technique for clearing your mind of all extraneous thoughts so that you can concentrate on relaxing. It can help you sleep better and release tension.

Acupuncture uses a series of very thin needles at specific points of the body remote from the area of pain.

Cognitive interventions are used to modify the pain experience. They include

Attention diversion, which reduces the impact of pain by focusing on other things.

Refocusing, which is used to distract from pain; it includes switching to activities such as listening to music or reading to keep your mind off of pain.

Pain inoculation training, which involves preparing for the pain mentally before it occurs.

Massage can provide tremendous relief for tight muscles. For anyone with osteoporosis, it should be done under the supervision of a physical therapist to prevent fractures.

TENS stands for transcutaneous electrical nerve stimulation. TENS delivers low-frequency electric current from a small battery pack through electrodes placed on the skin. Some people get tremendous relief from TENS, while others get none.

CHAPTER EIGHT

QUESTIONS AND ANSWERS

Are there any natural remedies for osteoporosis?

Dr. Ross Trattler, a practicing naturopathic physician and author of Better Health Through Natural Healing, recommends the botanicals comfrey and horsetail for osteoporosis.[1] Honey bee pollen and chlorella also include many nutrients important to bone health. In addition, most health food stores sell acidophilus to aid digestion and increase calcium absorption. But, remember, never take herbs and roots without the advice of an experienced professional such as a licensed physician or nutritionist.

Are there any natural remedies for fractures?

According to Dr. Stephen Cummings and Dana Ullman, authors of Everybody's Guide to Homeopathic Medicine,

---

[1] Ross Trattler, Better Health Through Natural Healing, (New York: McGraw-Hill, 1985), p. 472.

homeopathic treatments can reduce pain, swelling, and shock after a fracture. They recommend taking Arnica or Eupatorium perfoliatum every three hours during the first two to three days. Symphytum, or comfrey, can be taken to aid healing after the initial pain and swelling have gone down.[2]

What are some recommendations for treating meno-pause that I would find at my local health food store and not at a pharmacy?

Herbs frequently used for menopause are ginseng and cohosh. However, if you cannot take estrogen, you should not try these. They can be dangerous. An excellent source for herbal remedies for menopause is Ourselves, Growing Older, by the Boston Women's Health Collective.[3]

What is the relationship between osteoporosis and osteoarthritis?

Technically both are classified as forms of arthritis. However, they are very different. Simply put, osteoar-

---

[2] Stephen Cummings and Dana Ullman, Everybody's Guide to Homeopathic Medicines, (Los Angeles: Tarcher, 1991), pp. 229-231.

[3] Paula Brown Doress, Diann Lastin Siegal, and The Midlife and Older Women Book Project, Ourselves, Growing Older, (New York: Simon and Schuster, 1987).

thritis affects the joints, whereas osteoporosis affects the bones. The major symptom of osteoarthritis is lost joint cartilage. This characteristic is distinctive and can be seen on an X ray. Soreness and loss of mobility are common. Osteoporosis is a condition in which bone mass decreases. The pain that accompanies osteoporosis is caused by fractures, not deteriorating joints.

If I have osteoporosis, does that mean that I will develop osteoarthritis?

Not necessarily, but both are associated with aging. In fact, virtually everyone over age 65 has some osteoarthritis. But osteoporosis is easier to prevent than is osteoarthritis and does not have to occur with aging.

My mother is 65 years old and has lost at least an inch in height in the last year. Should I try to persuade her to take estrogen? To see a doctor?

Yes! and Yes! Your mother should discuss hormone replacement therapy with a physician and, if she isn't already getting regular weight-bearing exercise, get started on a program of exercise to increase her bone density. Also, the fact that your mother has osteoporosis means that you also are at high risk. You should start preventive measures yourself, if you haven't already.

I walk a couple of miles every day to ward off os-
teoporosis, but have a hard time convincing my hus-
band that he should walk with me. He says, "Men
don't get osteoporosis." Please print something I
can give him to read that will convince him other-
wise.

Increasing numbers of men are developing osteoporosis, particularly those who:

- Have poor eating habits and/or an eating disorder.

- Diet and/or fast frequently.

- Are physically inactive.

- Are immobilized.

- Are endurance athletes.

- Are heavy cigarette smokers.

- Are heavy drinkers of alcohol.

- Are senior citizens.

- Have a medical condition such as small-bowel disease or take a medication such as steroids that block calcium absorption.

- Have decreasing levels of testosterone.

<u>If I follow your steps to osteoporosis prevention, will I gain weight?</u>

No, because, you will be eating healthy food and getting lots of calorie-burning exercise.

<u>Every time I try calcium supplements I develop gas. Do you have any suggestions?</u>

Try taking Tums-EX™. Take four tablets a day, unless you are postmenopausal and not on estrogen, in which case you should take five tablets. <u>However, watch out for calcium-containing antacids that contain aluminum.</u> They can block the absorption of calcium and lead to other problems.

APPENDIX

RESOURCES AND RECIPIES

WHO'S WHO IN OSTEOPOROSIS CARE

The following covers most of the health professionals you are likely to see throughout your treatment for osteoporosis.

Family physicians or internists will diagnosis and treat your disease. They should provide preventive care, do routine check-ups, and refer you to a surgeon when necessary or perform surgery themselves. Your physician should be board certified by the medical board covering his or her specialty.

Orthopedists specialize in medical treatment of the skeletal system and related areas such as joints and muscles. Your orthopedist should be board certified.

Orthopedic surgeons operate on and treat problems of the bones, joints, muscles, ligaments, and tendons. Your surgeon should be board certified.

Physiatrists are physicians trained in rehabilitation.

Nurses—registered nurses and licensed practical nurses—provide direct, skilled nursing services, supervise other caregivers, coordinate patient care with the physician, and train family and friends so they can maintain a medical program set up by a physician.

Homemaker/home health aides provide personal care in the home such as assistance in bathing, grooming, dressing, cooking, and cleaning under the supervision of a professional person.

Physical and occupational therapists can play an invaluable role in home health care for osteoporosis patients. Their magic often enables the osteoporosis sufferer to be more independent at home and have a higher quality of life. Physical therapists help people whose strength, ability to move, sensation, or range of motion is impaired. They may use exercise; heat, cold, or water therapy; or other treatments to control pain, strengthen muscles, and improve coordination.

Occupational therapists assist patients with handicaps to function more independently. They may also provide exercise programs; heat, cold, and whirlpool treatments to relieve pain; and hand splints and adaptive equipment to improve function and independence.

Both physical and occupational therapists can help correct problems with posture, movements, and resting

Mock Mayonnaise

½ cup nonfat or low-fat yogurt
2 tsps lemon juice
Dash of sugar
1 tsp Dijon mustard
Dash of regular or celery salt

   Combine ingredients. Use anywhere you would use mayonnaise. Mix with canned salmon for a high-calcium lunch.

Yogurt Topping for Fruit

1 cup plain nonfat or low-fat yogurt
1 to 2 tbsps sugar or equivalent sweetener
1 tsp vanilla or fruit extract
2 tsp chopped mint
Pinch of cinnamon (optional)

   Combine ingredients.

Feta Cheese Dressing

1 cup plain nonfat or low-fat yogurt
2 ounces feta cheese
1 garlic clove, minced
2 tbsps chopped parsley
2 tbsps chopped scallions
¼ tsp dried oregano

   Combine ingredients in a food processor or blender.

Cucumber Dressing

1 peeled cucumber

1½ cups nonfat cottage cheese

¼ cup plain low-fat or nonfat yogurt

¼ cup chopped onion or 2 green onions

1 tsp dill

Combine ingredients in a food processor or blender.

White Sauces

Make casseroles and creamed dishes with these recipes for high-calcium meals. For example, mix chopped cooked chicken or turkey in light white sauce and serve over a baked potato or rice. (For added taste and calcium, sprinkle grated cheese on the top and put briefly under a broiler to brown.)

Light White Sauce

1 tbsp margarine or butter

1 tbsp flour

1 cup skim milk

3 tbsps dry milk

⅛ tsp cayenne pepper

Combine and cook until lightly bubbling.

Mornay Sauce

1 cup white sauce (see above)
1 tbsp grated Parmesan
⅛ tsp nutmeg

   Combine and cook until lightly bubbling.

Salmon Recipes

Potato-Salmon Croquettes

4 cups cooked, diced potatoes
8 ounce can salmon, drained, bones saved
⅓ cup chopped green pepper
⅓ cup chopped red or yellow pepper
2 tbsps minced onion
1 tsp chopped parsley
1 egg or egg substitute equivalent
Canola oil

   Blend drained salmon in food processor to crush bones.
In a mixing bowl, combine potatoes, blended salmon, and
other ingredients and shape into patties. Fry in canola
oil until browned on all sides.

Salmon Mousse

1 envelope unflavored gelatin
¼ to ½ cup water
8 ounces canned salmon
½ cup plain low-fat or nonfat yogurt
2 tsps fresh chopped dill

2 tsps chopped parsley
1 tbsp chopped onion
1 tsp chopped chives
2 tsps lemon juice
Dash cayenne
Dash spiced pepper

Sprinkle gelatin over water and let stand for about 5 minutes. Heat gelatin until melted. Purée salmon and yogurt and transfer to bowl. Pour gelatin mixture into salmon. Combine remaining ingredients. Pour into greased mold or bowl and refrigerate until set.

Smoked Salmon Dip

8 oz. can salmon, bones saved
1 cup low-fat cream cheese
1½ cups nonfat cottage cheese
¼ cup minced onion or scallion
½ tsp liquid smoke
1 tbsp chopped parsley
1 or more teaspoons chopped chives

Combine ingredients in a food processor or blender.

Cheese Casseroles

Rice with Cheese

4 cups cooked rice (white or brown, or, if desired, include wild rice)
1 cup reduced-fat Cheddar or Swiss cheese

1 cup skim milk or evaporated skim milk

1 cup bread crumbs

4 tbsps butter or margarine (optional)

Pinch of pepper

Pinch of paprika

Pinch of salt

In a baking dish layer half the rice, half the cheese, and half the spices. Repeat. Pour milk over casserole, dot with butter or margarine, cover top with bread crumbs, and bake in a preheated 350° F oven for 45 minutes. Try adding chopped turkey or chicken, water chestnuts, peppers, or mushrooms.

Low-Guilt Macaroni and Cheese

½ pound cooked macaroni noodles

2 cups reduced-fat Mornay sauce (see above)

½ cup grated reduced-fat Cheddar cheese

½ cup bread crumbs

¼ cup chopped pimento (optional)

¼ cup chopped onion, sauteed lightly (optional)

Mix macaroni and cheese sauce in a casserole dish. Sprinkle cheese over top and top with bread crumbs. Bake uncovered about 30 minutes in a preheated 375° F oven.

Stuffed Manicotti

2 cups low-fat cottage cheese

1 egg or egg equivalent

2 tbsps parsley or chopped cooked spinach

4 tbsps grated Parmesan cheese

¼ tsp nutmeg
¼ tsp salt
¼ tsp pepper
¼ tsp nutmeg

Mix cheese with other ingredients and stuff manicotti with mixture. Cover with marinara sauce of your choice or reduced-fat cheese sauce (see above) and bake in a preheated 375° F oven for 1 hour.

Potato-Leek Pie

1½ large baking potatoes, sliced
1 pound leeks, scrubbed and sliced
½ cup chicken or vegetable broth
2 tbsps chopped parsley
½ cup part-skim mozzarella cheese
Dash celery salt
Dash paprika

Boil potatoes until tender. Drain. Cook the leeks in stock until tender. Drain. Combine potatoes and leeks in layers in a well-greased casserole. Sprinkle parsley and spices over top and cover with cheese. Bake for half an hour in a preheated 325° F oven.

Broccoli Cheese Custard

2 cups chopped cooked broccoli, well drained
¾ cup grated reduced-fat Cheddar cheese
2 eggs or equivalent egg substitute
1½ cups evaporated skim milk
¼ tsp celery salt

¼ tsp pepper

Pinch nutmeg

Put broccoli in casserole and top with cheese. Beat eggs or egg equivalent with milk and spices and stir into mixture. Put enough water in a pan to cover one-half to three-fourths of sides of baking dish and put dish in pan. Bake in a preheated 350° F oven until set, about 45 minutes.

<u>Cheese Bread</u>

1 cup pastry flour

1 cup all-purpose flour

½ tsp baking soda

1½ tsps baking powder

2 tsps dry mustard

1½ to 2 cups low-fat Cheddar cheese, grated

2 eggs or equivalent

1 cup buttermilk

¼ cup canola oil

2 or 3 tbsps fresh chopped herbs such as basil or parsley
   (optional)

Sift flour, baking soda, baking powder, and mustard. Mix in cheese. In a separate bowl beat eggs, buttermilk, and oil until blended. Add to flour mixture and mix well. Pour into well-greased bread pan and bake in a preheated 375° F oven for 45 minutes. Serve with hot pepper jelly if available.

Desserts

Fruit Sherbert

2 cups berries or sliced fruit such as peaches,
    blueberries, or strawberries
½ cup nonfat or low-fat frozen yogurt
⅙ cup sugar or equivalent artificial sweetener
1 tsp vanilla or fruit extract
2 egg whites
Pinch nutmeg
Pinch cinnamon or pumpkin pie seasoning

Blend all ingredients except egg whites in food processor. Beat egg whites until stiff. Fold egg whites gently into other ingredients. Freeze. (Thaw slightly before serving.)

New Age Gelatin

1 package fruit-flavored gelatin
1 cup plain frozen yogurt
1 cup blended fruit

Prepare gelatin until slightly jelled; fold in yogurt and blended fruit.

GLOSSARY

Absorption   The uptake of nutrients by the
                        body.

Amenorrhea   The absence of menstrual flow
                        during the childbearing years.

Analgesic   A medication used to relieve pain.

Anorexia nervosa   An eating disorder that results in
                        malnutrition.

Bisphosphonates   Chemical compounds that stop bone
                        demolition.

Bone mass   The amount of bony material in
                        bone. Bone mass tests measure the
                        presence of osteoporosis.

Bone remodeling   A continuous renewal process that
                        the bones go through in which
                        small amounts of old bone are
                        taken away and new bone is added.

Bone resorption   The process by which small amounts
                        of old bone are broken down and
                        removed.

Bone turnover   The rate at which old bone is
                    demolished and new bone is recon-
                    structed.

Calcitonin   A hormone that inhibits bone re-
                    sorption.

Calcium   An element essential for normal
                    body development and maintenance.

Colles' fractures   Wrist fractures in the lower part
                    of a bone called the radius. Such
                    fractures usually happen as a
                    result of trying to break a fall.

Compact bone   One of two types of bone that is
                    nearly solid. Also called cortical
                    bone.

Compression
fractures   Wedge-shaped fractures of the ver-
                    tebrae.

Cortical bone   See compact bone.

Endometrium   The mucous membrane that lines the
                    uterus.

Estrogen   A female hormone.

Estrogen replacement
therapy (ERT)

Treatment in which estrogen is taken, often along with other hormones, to relieve symptoms of menopause, including development of osteoporosis.

Femur

The thigh bone. A long bone between the hip and the knee.

Fracture

Breakage or cracking of a bone.

Hormone replacement
therapy (HRT)

The addition of progestin to ERT. The progestin reduces the risk of endometrial cancer.

Hormones

Substances produced by the adrenal glands, ovaries, and other parts of the body. They influence organs and tissues.

Menopause

The period in a woman's life that follows the last menstrual period. It is accompanied by a reduction in estrogen.

Osteoblasts

Cells that construct new bone.

Osteoclasts

Cells that demolish old bone.

Osteocytes	Maintenance cells in bones.
Osteoporosis	A condition in which bones lose calcium and, consequently, break easily.
Ovaries	Two small organs located on each side of the utereus. The ovaries produce the hormones estrogen and progesterone.
Peak bone mass	The point at which bones are as strong and dense as they will ever be.
Photon	A unit of electromagnetic energy that is absorbed at a different rate by bone than other body tissues.
Progesterone	A female hormone produced in the ovaries.
Progestin	A synthetic form of progesterone.
Rickets	A condition caused by lack of vitamin D.
Risk factors	Factors that make individuals susceptible to development of a medical condition.

Spongy bone

A type of bone that is filled with holes and looks like a sponge. Spongy bones makes up the inside of bones. Also called trabecular bone.

Trabecular bone

See spongy bone.

Vertebrae

The 33 bones of the backbone or spine.

Vitamin D

A vitamin that aids in calcium absorption.

ORGANIZATIONS

National Osteoporosis Foundation (NOF)
Suite 602, Dept. J
2100 M Street N.W.
Washington, DC 20037-1207
(202) 223-2226

The National Osteoporosis Foundation is dedicated to finding answers to help you overcome osteoporosis. Membership in the organization provides you with self-help information, a quarterly newsletter, the latest medical facts, and free education materials. The NOF staff is extremely well informed and helpful to consumers.

The National Osteoporosis Foundation toll-free number is 1-800-223-9994. Operators answer questions about osteoporosis. Callers receive a 22-page brochure "Stand Up to Osteoporosis."

National Institute of Arthritis and Musculoskeletal and Skin Diseases (NIAMS)
Information Office
Building 31, Room B2B15
9000 Rockville Pike
Bethesda, MD 20892
(301) 496-8188

NIAMS is part of the National Institutes of Health. It is the federal government's principal agency for research on a number of arthritis-related diseases including osteoporosis. A variety of free publications about osteoporosis are available through the Institute by sending a postcard to the address given.

Calcium Information Center
Cornell University Medical Center
(800) 321-2681

Call the information center for the latest information on calcium and osteoporosis.

<u>Abledata</u>

National Rehabilitation Information Center

Catholic University of America

4407 8th Street N.E.

Washington, D.C. 20017-2299

(800) 34-NARIC

Abledata has a database of assistive devices, useful for those with advanced osteoporosis.

<u>American Academy of Orthopaedic Surgeons</u>

6300 River Road

Rosemont, IL 60018

(708) 823-7186

Contact the Academy to locate board-certified orthopaedic surgeons in your community.

<u>American College of Surgeons</u>

55 East Erie Street

Chicago, IL 60611

(313) 664-4050

Contact the College to locate board-certified surgeons in your community.